Practical and easy to use, this book is an effective resource for people who want to avoid the health problems caused by unmanaged long-term stress.

—DON COLBERT, MD
NEW YORK TIMES BEST-SELLING AUTHOR OF *THE SEVEN PILLARS OF HEALTH* AND THE BIBLE CURE SERIES

In this volume Dr. Mike Ronsisvalle offers classic, time-tested strategies to help those struggling with anxiety and stress. If implemented regularly, these strategies will help you to "transform your mind" and experience God's peace. If you or someone you love is over-stressed, this book will help.

—C. JEFFREY TERRELL, PHD
PSYCHOLOGIST AND PRESIDENT OF RICHMONT
GRADUATE UNIVERSITY

This thought-provoking, inspirational book is a thorough account of how stress can be successfully managed on a daily basis. It is a wonderfully useful tool that is user-friendly and hope-filled. With a refreshingly witty style, Dr. Mike's *Stress Relief for Life* is a compelling read. If you read just one health and wellness book this year, let this be the book.

—AARON TABOR, MD
AUTHOR OF *FIGHT NOW* AND *DR. TABOR'S SLIM & BEAUTIFUL DIET* AND FOUNDER OF PHYSICIANS LABORATORIES

From the very first pages, I was hooked. Dr. Mike not only described my stress-filled life in detail; he then threw out a lifeline. I felt I was having coffee with a friend as he laid out a twenty-one-day plan in his intelligent yet likable style. It's practical, it's easy, and best of all, it's doable. *Stress Relief for Life* is not only a good idea, but it's also a great resource...one I plan on sharing with my friends.

—ANN MAINSE
HOST, *FULL CIRCLE* TV SHOW

I know from personal experience that the strategies for stress relief set forth by Dr. Ronsisvalle in this volume really work. Unlike many secular alternatives, the spiritual dimension of human life is fully considered. This book is filled with psychological wisdom, biblical insight, and practical advice that will help everybody.

—TIMOTHY GEORGE
FOUNDING DEAN OF BEESON DIVINITY SCHOOL OF SAMFORD UNIVERSITY AND THEOLOGICAL ADVISOR FOR *CHRISTIANITY TODAY*

stress
relief
for life

Practical solutions to help you
relax and live better

MIKE RONSISVALLE, PsyD

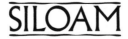

Most CHARISMA HOUSE BOOK GROUP products are available at special quantity discounts for bulk purchase for sales promotions, premiums, fund-raising, and educational needs. For details, write Charisma House Book Group, 600 Rinehart Road, Lake Mary, Florida 32746, or telephone (407) 333-0600.

STRESS RELIEF FOR LIFE by Michael Ronsisvalle, PsyD
Published by Siloam
Charisma Media/Charisma House Book Group
600 Rinehart Road
Lake Mary, Florida 32746
www.charismahouse.com

Cover design by Marvin Eans
Design Director: Bill Johnson

Visit the author's website at www.MyRealityOnline.com.

Library of Congress Cataloging-in-Publication Data:
Ronsisvalle, Mike.
  Stress relief for life / Mike Ronsisvalle.
     p. cm.
  Includes bibliographical references and index.
  ISBN 978-1-61638-357-2 (trade paper) -- ISBN 978-1-61638-432-6 (e-book) 1. Stress (Psychology) 2. Stress management. 3.

Relaxation. I. Title.
  BF575.S75R655 2011
  155.9'042--dc22

2011004630

First Edition

11 12 13 14 15 — 9 8 7 6 5 4 3 2 1
Printed in the United States of America

CONTENTS

Introduction 1

Day One
The Lowdown on Stress................................7

Day Two
It's a Matter of Time.................................. 17

Day Three
Take Time to Relax: Active Relaxation 23

Day Four
Take Time to Relax: Passive Relaxation...................... 33

Day Five
Dissect Your Stress 41

Day Six
Clue In to Your Thoughts and Feelings...................... 53

Day Seven
Challenge Your Stress-Inducing Thoughts.................. 61

Day Eight
Get to the Core of Your Stress: People Pleasing....... 69

Day Nine
**Get to the Core of Your Stress:
Performance and Control**.........................77

Day Ten
The Old Story 89

Day Eleven
Your New Story.................................... 101

Day Twelve
Your Personalized System for Stress Management...115

Day Thirteen
  Pursue Stress?... 133
Day Fourteen
  The Power of Exercise 141
Day Fifteen
  Make Room for Margin................................ 151
Day Sixteen
  Do What You Love 163
Day Seventeen
  Cultivate Supportive Relationships 173
Day Eighteen
  Embrace Radical Change 185
Day Nineteen
  Confront Your Fears................................... 195
Day Twenty
  Trust God's Power in Your Life 205
Day Twenty-One
  Whatever You Do, Don't Quit 215
  Conclusion... 223
  Notes... 225
  Selected Bibliography................................ 227
  Index 229

INTRODUCTION

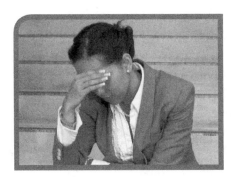

THE SIGNS ARE all around us, in the chatter you hear in almost any living room, office, classroom, or coffeehouse:

- "I can't believe it's 6:30 p.m. already, and I'm not done with this proposal."

- "Would you just shut up and listen to me? I'm not going to sit here and argue with you all night."

- "Honey, I think Jenny is having sex with her boyfriend. I found birth control pills in her closet."

- "I've got mail...again?"

- "Twelve more American soldiers were killed today at the hands of a suicide bomber..."

- "Mom, I am not too young to wear a miniskirt!"

- "The baby is up again, and I've got to make a presentation tomorrow morning."

- "I just can't take it anymore!"

Life is more complicated than ever before, and people are overwhelmed and overstressed. Just look around. People are pulsating in the pressure cooker of unbridled expectations at work and at home. Companies now pride themselves on their ability to do more with less manpower. They call it downsizing; everyone else calls it torture. And we can't find a respite at home because the simplicity of family life has been replaced with what can be described only as chaotic over-scheduling. Children are juggling soccer games, dance classes, church activities, and tutoring—all in the same day.

Despite its modern advancements, the twenty-first century has made our lives more complex. Family configurations are morphing rapidly, and technology is only adding to the stress it was supposed to eliminate. Twenty-four-hour, five-hundred-channel TV access; unlimited cell phone service; and ever-present wireless Internet connections make life exciting but extremely exhausting. As a society, we are literally coming apart at the seams as we become victims of our own impossible schedules and chronically disconnected relationships. And it seems as if there is no end in sight.

During my training as a clinical psychologist, I was encouraged to look for the underlying issues behind a person's "presenting problem" of stress. Was it a troubled childhood? How about some significant trauma suffered earlier in life or a current interpersonal crisis? As it turns out, much of my practical experience in counseling tells me that the presenting problem underneath stress often involves difficulty managing what we consider normal, everyday life.

It's Not Supposed to Be This Way!

One of my graduate school professors at Wheaton College, Dr. Mark McMinn, had a very practical way of explaining why so many people get chronically stressed. I'll paraphrase his understanding of the root cause of stress with this illustration from the 1991 film *Grand Canyon*.[1]

In the movie, a young man played by Kevin Kline drives down a crowded interstate in Los Angeles. As he surveys what seems like miles of brake lights ahead of him, he makes a snap decision to pull off the highway and take the back roads to avoid the congestion. After some time, it becomes apparent that he is lost. He finds himself driving his late-model BMW through the slums of LA when the unthinkable happens: he has car trouble. His Beamer creeps to a stop on the side of the road, and he immediately picks up his cell phone and calls for a tow truck.

Before long his car is surrounded by what looks like a group of gang members, and what the man fears begins to unfold. The gang members pull him from his car and start to beat him up. The situation doesn't look good at all for the young driver until his tow truck arrives. Out from the cab jumps a strapping driver played by Danny Glover, who promptly pulls the gang leader aside.

Glover's character looks this young gang leader in the eyes and says something along these lines: "Look, I'm here to do my job. I'm just a tow truck driver, and my job is to help this guy get his car back home. And this guy"—Glover points to the driver of the BMW—"he's just trying to get home. But here we are, and you guys are about to beat the fool out of this guy. This isn't right. It's just not supposed to be this way."[2]

It's just not supposed to be this way. Every time I watch *Grand Canyon* I'm shocked at how profound this statement is. Amazingly, it carries great theological weight. We are not supposed to be so stressed. Life shouldn't feel so chaotic for so many people. God never intended this, but our world is just broken. What Glover's character confronts that day in Los Angeles and what we experience every day in our stress-filled lives is a result of the brokenness of our world.

Our world is characterized by pain, marred by sin, and in many ways we are broken people. The question is, What are we to do with our brokenness? Do we embrace it? Do we live with our stress and make the best of it? I don't think so! God has a plan to heal the brokenness of our lives in general and the brokenness of our own personal world in particular. He hasn't left us hanging in the balance, and He has indeed provided strategies that can help us overcome chronic stress and experience a life filled with peace.

That's where *Stress Relief for Life* comes in. This program is designed to take you from the brokenness of stress to the beauty of a peace that passes all understanding. For the next twenty-one days you will be exposed to information about how to live a less-stressed life, but more importantly, you will learn practical skills that you can implement in any situation to get relief from the pressure cooker of your life.

This program is not a dissertation on the theoretical

underpinnings of stress in general. Instead we will focus on what to do in the unique and specific situations that create chronic stress in your life. Each day you will be given assignments that will help you identify the sources of your stress and discover new ways to respond to those triggers.

I've also made two audio CDs available for download at www.myrealityonline.com that will guide you through active and passive progressive relaxation. If you're not technologically savvy, don't worry. I will explain these relaxation techniques in detail on days two and three. Whether you read through the relaxation process or follow the CDs, progressive relaxation will play a critical role in helping you de-stress, so I will ask you to practice one of these techniques daily.

The Stress Relief for Life program is simple, practical, and based on solid research regarding the most effective techniques for managing stress. The plan works, but only if you take the time to implement it. I realize that if you had a lot of time on your hands, you probably wouldn't be stressed. But if you are motivated to spend thirty minutes each day reading the material, completing the assignments, and implementing the stress-management skills in your life, you will be considerably less stressed in twenty-one days.

It is important to note that this program will not eliminate stress from your life. It's unrealistic to think that you can live without stress because we all need a little stress to help motivate us. However, it is realistic to eradicate your *chronic* stress and begin to live a life that feels totally different. You can experience the kind of life God intended—one that is filled with His peace even in the midst of the most stressful situations. So, are you ready to begin?

Day One

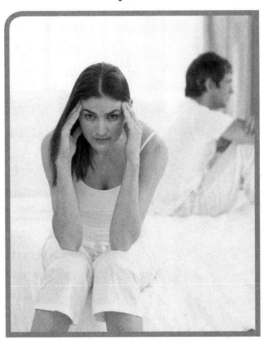

THE LOWDOWN ON STRESS

CONGRATULATIONS! BY EMBARKING on this twenty-one-day program, you have taken an important first step toward living a less-stressed life. But there's real work to be done if you want to see lasting change. First, you must understand what stress is and what impact it is having on your life.

People often think of stress as pressure at work, a demanding boss, a sick child, or rush-hour traffic. All of these may be triggers to stress, but stress is actually the body's reaction to situations such as these. Stress is the body's fight-or-flight response, which is driven by adrenaline and other stress hormones that are released when we perceive a situation as threatening. When we start to feel stressed-out, we are actually tuning in to some physical changes that occur in our bodies as a result of the stress hormones, including increased heart rate and blood

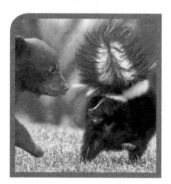

pressure, faster breathing, muscle tension, dilated pupils, dry mouth, and elevated blood sugar.

By definition, stress is the state of increased physical arousal necessary for a living being to defend itself in time of danger. Let me show you how this plays out in the real world. I grew up in a rural part of Merritt Island, Florida. Our house was surrounded by wooded areas and orange groves, and I had many run-ins with a multitude of wild animals, including raccoons, opossums, wild hogs, and even alligators.

Of all the lessons I learned while growing up in this environment, the most important was that you never corner a wild animal. If you ever do, the fight-or-flight response will cause the animal to rear up and brace for a confrontation. It's quite a scary sight to see an animal that feels threatened.

As strange as it may sound, you are much like those wild animals I encountered growing up. When you engage an environment that you perceive as threatening or overwhelming, your stress hormones release a tremendous amount of energy in your body. This stress reaction is in your mind and body, not "out there" in the situation or environment. Dr. Philip Eichling, a specialist in sleep medicine, defines stress as "the mind's interpretation of an event in a way that causes characteristic physical effects."[1] Basically, stress is the body's response to situations that we perceive or interpret as threatening, dangerous, overwhelming, or "impossible." It is brought on by the way we think about the events in our lives.

Just like in those wild animals out on Merritt Island, the stress response in our bodies gives us the strength and energy to either engage the fight or run away from danger. One problem is that it is rarely appropriate for us to unleash all the strength and energy these stress hormones release. Think about it: we can't just run out of the room and down the hall when we are asked a tough question during the morning staff meeting. The result is that our bodies go into a state of high energy when we perceive we are in a stressful or threatening environment, but there is usually no place for that energy to go. I've worked with many patients struggling to manage their stress whose bodies remained in a state of arousal for hours or even days at a time.

This, and even less extreme responses to chronic stress, can be devastating on our bodies. The National Institute for

Occupational Safety and Health finds that stress-related ailments cost companies about $200 billion a year in increased absenteeism, tardiness, and the loss of talented workers. Between 70 and 90 percent of employee hospital visits are

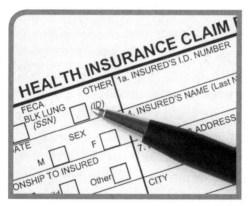

linked to stress, and as much as 90 percent of all visits to family doctors are for reasons related to stress.[2]

In a nutshell, stress is the number one health problem at work and at home. Stress-related physical symptoms include headaches, insomnia, muscle aches and stiffness (especially in the neck, shoulders, and lower back), heart palpitations, chest pains, abdominal cramps, nausea, trembling, cold extremities, flushing or sweating, and frequent colds. It is important to note that one of the most common symptoms of chronic stress is fatigue, which we tend to ignore.

In addition to its negative physical consequences, stress can manifest itself in a number of other areas of our functioning:

- Emotionally. Stress can cause us to feel "uneven" emotionally. This lack of emotional stability can feel like anxiety, nervousness, depression, anger, frustration, worry, fear, irritability, impatience, and short temper.

- Mentally. Symptoms of stress include a decrease in concentration and memory, indecisiveness, the mind racing or going blank, confusion, and loss of a sense of humor.

- Behaviorally. It probably comes as no surprise that chronic stress has a tremendous impact upon our behaviors. Stress-driven behaviors include pacing, fidgeting, nervous habits (nail biting and foot tapping), increased eating, smoking, drinking, crying, yelling, swearing, blaming, and even throwing or hitting things.

- Relationally. Of all the areas stress impacts, it might take its most stealth-like toll on our relationships. Have you ever come home and yelled at your kids after a hard day at work? Or have you ever had an unusually hard day at the office after a fight with your spouse? Although we don't always connect these dots, the extra energy we get from stress usually seeps out as anger in our relationships.

- Spiritually. Positive and healthy spirituality is associated with a peace that exceeds human understanding. When we have a stress-filled life, our spiritual peace begins to fade because we end up exchanging a focus on the eternal for a preoccupation with our stress triggers. The bottom line is that chronic stress and true connectedness with God fight against each other.

I've included two exercises at the end of today's reading to help you determine how stress is affecting your life. The Stress Assessment will give you an idea of whether you have more stress-inducing experiences or encounter more stressful environments than most. And the Effects of Stress exercise will help you gain insight into how stress is impacting your physical, emotional, relational, and spiritual life. These exercises not only will help you determine your stress level, but they also will allow you to measure your progress as you move toward a less-stressed life.

Assignment

- Complete the Stress Assessment.
- Complete the Effects of Stress worksheet.

ASSESS YOUR STRESS LEVEL

This assessment was designed several years ago by psychiatrists Thomas Holmes and Richard Rahe, who were doing research in the area of stress management.[3] Although some people who experience chronic stress don't produce high scores on this measure (you'll find out why as you go through this program), it provides a gauge to determine whether or not you are confronting situations that are easy to interpret as stressful or overwhelming. Accordingly, your "score" on this assessment should be used only as a guideline for potential stress-inducing situations.

To measure your stress level for the year, mark every life event that applies to you and then add up your points. Three hundred points is regarded as a danger zone because those who score above that level have a 90 percent chance of experiencing a major health problem as a result of their stress.

Life Event	Value	Life Event	Value
Death of spouse	100	Son or daughter leaving home	29
Divorce	73	Trouble with in-laws	29
Marital separation	65	Outstanding personal achievement	29
Jail term	63	Spouse begins or stops work	26
Death of close family member	63	Begin or end school	26
Personal injury or illness	53	Change in living conditions	25
Marriage	50	Revisions of personal habits	24
Fired at work	47	Trouble with boss	23

Life Event	Value	Life Event	Value
Marital reconciliation	45	Change in work hours or conditions	20
Retirement	45	Change in residence	20
Change in health of family member	44	Change in schools	20
Pregnancy	40	Change in recreational habits	19
Sex difficulties	39	Change in church activities	19
Gain of new family member	39	Change in social activities	18
Business readjustment	39	Mortgage or loan of less than $100,000	17
Change in financial state	38	Change in sleeping habits	16
Death of a close friend	37	Change in eating habits	15
Change to a different line of work	36	Change in number of family gatherings	15
Change in number of arguments with spouse	35	Vacation	13
Mortgage or loan over $100,000	31	Christmas	12
Foreclosure of mortgage or loan	30	Minor violations of the law	11
Change in responsibilities at work	29	**TOTAL POINTS**	

THE EFFECTS OF STRESS

Stress can have a devastating impact upon several areas of your life. The problem is that most people never stop to examine just how destructive their stress really is. Think about how stress has affected your life in the following areas in order to gain insight into how stress is impacting you negatively. Write your answers in the spaces provided.

Your physical health

_____

_____

_____

_____

Your relationships

_____

_____

_____

_____

Your emotional and mental health

_____

_____

_____

_____

Your spiritual health

_____

_____

_____

_____

Your professional life

_____

_____

_____

_____

Day Two

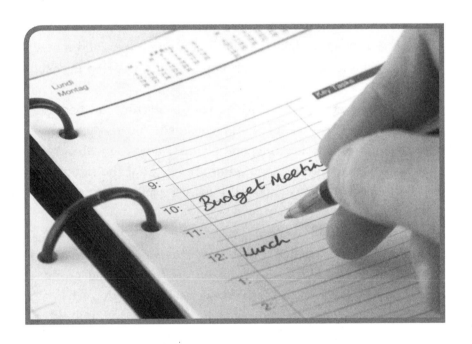

IT'S A MATTER OF TIME

ARE YOU READY to surrender your stress? As I said yesterday, if you think you're ready to embark on a new life that is less stressed, you are going to have to commit to real behavior change. Interestingly enough, one of the hardest behavior changes you will make is creating time to read this book, complete the exercises, and implement the skills in your everyday life. Being less stressed is, generally speaking, all about time: creating more time (on the job, at home, and with friends) to do the things that will lead to less stress and more peace. Making time for this program is your first step in that process.

How do you do this? How do you create time to manage your stress if you are already overscheduled? You must visit the next nineteen days mentally and plan out how you will create the time to complete this program. If you want the future to be different, you must make things different in the present. You have to *make* time—now.

I was in a situation similar to the one you may be in right now when I started putting together this stress-management program. I was already working on another writing project and heavily involved in a private counseling practice. I had a

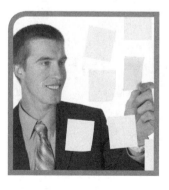

very real passion to communicate the information contained in this program to a broad audience, but I had little time to put it all together.

After much deliberation about how to fit another project on my plate, I made a decision to make time right then and there. I decided to cut back my ten-hour workday by 10 percent to end an hour earlier. At first I was concerned that my productivity would decrease, but I found that, overall, I was getting just as much done in nine hours at the office as I had completed within ten hours. Instead of becoming less productive, I found that I was more satisfied and engaged at the office because I was doing something I was passionate about. I changed how I worked, but not how much work I got done.

Now, don't get me wrong: surrendering a portion of my day was not without its challenges. I didn't return every phone call, and I had to cut down on the number of appointments I set. But in the end, I created an hour every day in which to engage something I really believed in.

This principle will work for you as well as you carve out time to complete the Stress Relief for Life program. Because this program is designed to take thirty minutes a day, including reading and assigned exercises, you might be able to cut down your workday by only 5 percent to free up enough time. If cutting down your workday or daily responsibilities is not possible, then identify a specific time of the day that you could use to complete the program. Can you wake up thirty minutes earlier? How about staying up thirty minutes later? Could you devote thirty minutes at lunchtime to completing these exercises?

Whatever you decide to do, it is important to set aside time every day (preferably at the same time of day) if you are determined to live a less-stressed life. Instead of a loss of productivity, you will find that you will be more satisfied and engaged in your day because you are doing something that is helping you manage your stress. In the end, you will probably find that learning to handle stress effectively will help increase your productivity.

Because this program builds on itself, I would love to see you complete it within the twenty-one-day schedule. This will ensure that you get the most out of the program and reap the benefits quickly. In order to accomplish this, you must begin scheduling your thirty-minute Stress Relief sessions now.

To help you think through which part of your day will work best for the sessions, it will be beneficial for you to complete the Creating a Stress-Free Zone worksheet. After you decide on a time, commit to follow through with the program every day. Protecting this time is very important because maintaining consistency with this program is the first step toward a future that is less stressed.

Assignment

- Complete the Creating a Stress-Free Zone exercise.

CREATING A STRESS-FREE ZONE

Finding time to complete the Stress Relief for Life program is essential to its effectiveness. Therefore it is critical that you decide in advance when you will read the material and complete the exercises. Remember, if you want the future to be different, you must make things different in the present. Follow the steps below to create a consistent time each day for your Stress Relief session.

DETERMINE WHEN YOU WILL COMPLETE THE STRESS RELIEF SESSIONS.

During which time of the day do you function best? Some people are more aware during the wee hours of the morning. Others function better at night. Choose a time of day in which you are more likely to be energized and able to focus on mentally and emotionally challenging material.

Many people experience success with this program when they build it into their workday. Because the reading and exercises are designed to take about thirty minutes each day, perhaps you can cut down your workday by 5 to 10 percent in order to make the room in your schedule.

> I will complete my Stress Relief sessions *during the week* at the following time:
>
> _____ o'clock to _____ o'clock
>
> I will complete my Stress Relief sessions *on the weekend* at the following time:
>
> _____ o'clock to _____ o'clock

DETERMINE WHERE YOU WILL COMPLETE THE STRESS RELIEF SESSIONS.

Will you complete the program at work? At home? At school? Become intentional about succeeding in this program by choosing an environment that will allow you to focus exclusively on your session.

I will complete my Stress Relief sessions *during the week* at the following location:

_____

I will complete my Stress Relief sessions *on the weekend* at the following location:

_____

WHAT COULD POTENTIALLY KEEP YOU FROM FOLLOWING THROUGH WITH THE STRESS RELIEF SESSIONS?

Will it be unexpected meetings at the office? How about makeup soccer games for the kids? If you want to complete your sessions, it is vitally important that you anticipate what schedule conflicts might occur and determine how you will respond to those interruptions.

Potential Block	Response
1.	1.
2.	2.
3.	3.
4.	4.
5.	5.

Day Three

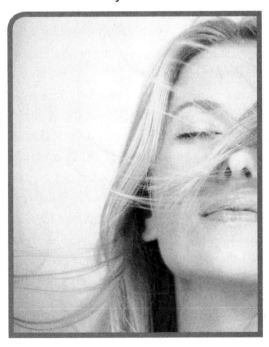

TAKE TIME TO RELAX: ACTIVE RELAXATION

WHAT WOULD YOU do to release a little stress? Ride a motorcycle at 110 miles an hour down the interstate? That's too dangerous. Join in a group break dance at the office? That's a bit dated. How about vigorously shaking your arms and legs in your family room? That might make your family wonder if they should call 911. While these activities might relieve some of your stress, they won't do much to help you attain the most important element of a less-stressed life—relaxation.

That sounds simple enough, doesn't it? Just relax. Having a nice dinner out seems relaxing. How about sitting down on the couch to watch your favorite movie? That also sounds relaxing to me. But the interesting thing about relaxation is

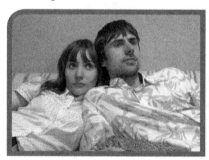

that most of us don't know how to do it very well. That night out for dinner usually involves a great deal of effort, including taking a shower, choosing an outfit, driving to the restaurant, and paying way too much for dinner. That favorite movie? It probably induces some pretty significant emotion inside of you, and significant emotion is not very consistent with true relaxation.

Researchers have noticed the inconsistency between what we like to do and what is actually relaxing. Because stress starts with a physiological arousal that is based on our perception of a situation as overwhelming, these same researchers have explored what kind of experiences actually lead to a truly relaxed physical state. You might be shocked to discover what the researchers found. Dinner, a movie, or even a good night's sleep won't effectively combat the physical arousal caused by stress.

One of the only activities that actually counteracts the physical effects of stress on the body is called progressive relaxation.[1] This technique is pretty simple. Basically, progressive relaxation is a process in which you intentionally and systematically relax every major muscle group in your body. While you are focusing on relaxing your muscles, you breathe deeply and steadily from your diaphragm. Although there are variations of progressive relaxation, this pretty much sums it up: you breathe and relax your muscles.

Researchers have consistently found that this kind of relaxation fights the adrenaline and other stress hormones that wreak havoc on you physiologically when you are under stress. Progressive relaxation releases other hormones that fight and win the battle for control of your body. And as I mentioned earlier, progressive relaxation actually relaxes your body more than sleep does. In fact, you can sleep for nine or ten hours and still not experience the kind of physical relaxation that progressive relaxation produces. That's why many people live in a chronic state of stress—they wake up just as stressed as they were when they went to bed because they are not intentionally and systematically relaxing their bodies.

The beautiful part about progressive relaxation is that it teaches you how to take the edge off your body's stress reaction in a very short period of time. I am going to ask you to practice progressive relaxation for twenty minutes every day until the Stress Relief for Life program is complete. If you comply with the program and are diligent about practicing progressive relaxation daily, at the end of the twenty-one days you will be able to create a more relaxed state in just two or three minutes. Some people can even gain a significant measure of relaxation in just sixty seconds.

Before you get all excited, let me put this into some perspective. Progressive relaxation is like riding a bicycle. At first it is very difficult to do. You might fall occasionally. You might even be convinced that you will never learn how to do it. But just like a child who keeps practicing on his bike, when you get it, you'll have it forever. You will spend several hours through the rest of this program learning how to systematically and intentionally relax your body. And when you learn how to relax, you'll have this skill forever.

It's Your Turn

Let's get started. Progressive relaxation can be achieved using either active relaxation techniques or passive relaxation techniques. You won't know which works best for you until you try them both. We'll start with active relaxation techniques today. I have included an exercise at the end of today's reading that will walk you through roughly twenty minutes of active relaxation. These steps also can be found on CD One, which is available for download at www.myrealityonline.com.

Before you begin the process of active relaxation, let me give you some quick pointers. Breathing correctly is an incredibly important part of progressive relaxation in general and active relaxation in particular; therefore, when you start your deep breathing, make sure that you are breathing from your diaphragm, not your chest. This means you will want to breathe from the deepest part of your stomach rather than taking breaths that are quick and shallow.

One method to help you breathe from your diaphragm is what I call the two-hand technique. It's so easy you can practice it now. Put one hand on your chest and the other on your stomach. Now take a deep breath. Which hand moved, the one on your stomach or your chest? If the hand on your chest moved up and down or in and out, you took a shallow breath, and that will not work well with progressive relaxation. Your goal is to take deep breaths that will make the hand on your stomach go in and out while the hand on your chest stays still.

As you follow the instructions for active relaxation, also stay mindful of how you flex each individual muscle group. You will start with your hands and arms, then move through every major muscle group until you have relaxed your entire body. It is important to flex each muscle group hard enough for you to experience some tension but not so hard that it is painful.

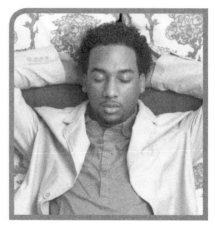

For instance, if I asked you to ball your hand into a fist and squeeze it tightly, you'd want to make sure you were squeezing tightly enough to create tension but not so tightly that your hand was in actual pain. When I teach clients active relaxation at my private practice, sometimes they squeeze their fists so hard they literally shake. This isn't necessary, and it might even prevent relaxation.

Now you are ready to begin. You can spend the rest of your time today practicing active relaxation using the guide I've included or the downloadable CD. If you plan to use the written instructions, you may find it helpful to have someone read them aloud to you so you can complete the process without interruption. In time you will be able to practice active relaxation without assistance. You might not fully understand it right now, but you are building skills that will ultimately lead you to a less-stressed life. Now, go relax.

Assignment

- Practice active relaxation for twenty minutes using CD One or the guide at the end of today's reading.

ACTIVE RELAXATION EXERCISE

Get as comfortable as you possibly can. You may even want to lie down on a couch or a bed. Close your eyes to shut the world out, and begin to take deep breaths in and out. Remember to breathe from the deepest part of your stomach and avoid taking breaths from your chest that are shallow and quick.

Count to three slowly as you breathe in. Hold the breath, then breathe out as you slowly count to three. Repeat the process several more times. You'll want to continue taking these kinds of deep breaths through the entire process of active relaxation.

Now, focus your attention on your hands and make a fist. As you continue to take deep breaths in and out, squeeze your fists rather tightly. Hold the tension in your hands for a count of three, then release your fist and let your hands relax and feel soft. Notice the difference between the tension of the clenched fist and the feeling of your hand at rest. Think to yourself, "My hands are starting to feel soft and relaxed."

Switch your focus from your hands to your forearms. Flex the muscles in your forearms, and hold it for a count of three. Say quietly to yourself, "My forearms feel soft and extremely heavy." Continue to let your forearms feel heavy, soft, and relaxed as you breathe in and out.

Next, turn your attention to your biceps. Focus in on your stress and begin to let the tension go to your biceps. As you breathe deeply, flex those bicep muscles for a count of three. Say quietly, "My biceps are soft, relaxed, and feeling extremely heavy. As a matter-of-fact, my arms feel heavy." As you breathe deeply from your abdomen, I want you to feel your arms becoming heavy as you focus all your attention on your arms.

Now move your focus from your arms to your face. Start with your forehead, because many people carry their stress in their foreheads. I want you to lift your eyebrows up as high as they can go. That will flex the muscles in your forehead. Hold it for a count of three, then release the tension. Let the muscles in your forehead relax. Tell yourself your forehead feels extremely soft, relaxed, pliable, and heavy. As you continue to breathe deeply, I want you to let your forehead feel heavy. Let your forehead feel soft.

Next, switch your attention from your forehead to your mouth. Open your mouth as wide as you possibly can. This will flex the muscles in your entire face. I want you to say to yourself, "My entire face feels soft and relaxed." As you continue to breathe deeply, I want you to let your entire face feel soft, relaxed, and pliable.

From your face, let's move down to your shoulders. I want you to notice any tension in your shoulders and begin to let it go. Flex the muscles in your shoulders by trying to touch your ears with your shoulders. Hold the position for the count of three. Notice the difference between the tension in your shoulders and the relaxation you're feeling now. Tell yourself that your shoulders feel soft and relaxed; your shoulders feel pliable and heavy.

Let's try that again. The shoulders are extremely important because a lot of people carry stress in their shoulders. Focus all your attention on your shoulders, and try to touch your ears with your shoulders. Hold the pose for the count of three, then let go. Tell yourself, "My shoulders are soft and relaxed and pliable. My shoulders feel extremely heavy." As you continue to breathe deeply from the diaphragm, I want you to let your shoulders feel heavy, pliable, and relaxed.

Now switch your focus from your shoulders to your stomach. Flex the muscles in your stomach, holding that position for the count of three. Let the muscles in your stomach feel incredibly relaxed, and notice the difference between the feeling of tension and that of relaxation. As you continue to breathe in and out, tell yourself that your stomach is starting to feel warm and soft.

Repeat the relaxation process for your stomach and abdomen. Flex the muscles in your abdomen, then let them go. As you continue to breathe deeply from your abdomen, I want you to let your abdomen feel incredibly relaxed. Just breathe in and breathe out. Tell yourself in your own head, "My stomach is feeling soft. It feels relaxed. It feels pliable." Let your stomach and your entire abdomen feel relaxed.

Now I want you to focus your attention on your entire upper body: your hands, your forearms, your biceps, all your facial muscles, and your abdomen. Let your entire upper body feel relaxed, soft, and pliable. As you continue to breathe deeply, I want you to let your entire upper body feel heavy. Notice any residual stress in your upper body. Continue to take deep breaths from your abdomen. Hold each breath for the count of three, then breathe out for a count of three. Tell yourself, "My entire upper body is feeling heavy."

Now you'll want to move your focus down to your hamstrings, which are the muscles from your knees to your waist. Contract those muscles by imagining that you're about to lift your heel and contract your hamstring. Feel the tension as you flex your hamstrings and hold them for the count of three. Say quietly, "My hamstrings, the entire upper part of my legs, are starting to feel relaxed and heavy."

Next, shift your attention down to your feet. Put your feet flat and raise your heels. This is going to flex your calf muscles. Hold this position for the count of three, then release it. Let your calf muscles feel incredibly relaxed. Tell yourself your calf muscles are starting to feel warm, pliable, and very heavy. Repeat this process with your calves once more, raising your heels to flex those muscles. Then relax them and allow your calves to feel warm and soft.

Now ball your feet up and keep the muscles contracted for the count of three. As you continue to breathe deeply, let your feet feel soft, relaxed, and pliable. Let your feet feel heavy and relaxed. Let your entire lower body—everything below your waist—feel heavy and relaxed.

Now I want you to scan your entire body for any signs of residual tension. Continue to take deep breaths, and think about the muscles in your hands and arms. They should feel relaxed and very warm. Your hands should feel heavy. The muscles in your forearm should feel soft and pliable. Tell yourself, "My forearms feel relaxed." The muscles in your biceps should feel loose and smooth. Let both arms feel extremely heavy. Say, "My biceps are extremely relaxed."

The muscles in your forehead and face should feel relaxed and warm. Tell yourself, "My face is entirely relaxed." The muscles in your shoulders should be very soft and pliable. Let your shoulders feel extremely heavy and loose, and say to yourself, "My shoulders are extremely heavy and relaxed." The muscles in your stomach should be calm. Let your stomach rise and fall slowly and rhythmically and say, "My stomach muscles are extremely relaxed."

The muscles in your hamstrings and upper legs should feel extremely loose. The muscles in your calves should feel extremely soft. Your feet should feel incredibly soft and loose. Say to yourself, "Everything below my waist is relaxed and heavy."

Now take a deep breath. Breathe in from your abdomen, and hold it for the count of three. Then exhale at the count of three. As you exhale, let any residual tension in your body drain away. Breathe deeper than before. As you breathe in and out, I want you to let your whole body feel heavy. Take several more deep breaths, then open your eyes.

Day Four

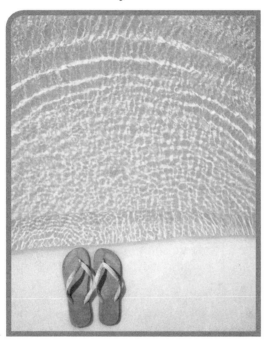

TAKE TIME TO RELAX:
PASSIVE RELAXATION

A LTHOUGH THE ACTIVE relaxation you read about yesterday will work for anyone, some people prefer a technique called passive relaxation. Both strategies work to produce the same relaxation response in your body, but passive relaxation accomplishes this through a less physical and more imaginative approach. In short, while active relaxation requires you to physically flex each muscle group, passive relaxation relies upon your ability to imagine each muscle group being systematically relaxed.

Because you won't be sure which approach works best for you until you try both, your assignment for today is to do just that: practice both active and passive relaxation. I've included an exercise to guide you through passive relaxation, but you can also practice this technique by downloading CD Two from www.myrealityonline.com. Make sure you spend at least twenty minutes completing the process.

After you complete passive relaxation, turn your attention back to yesterday's exercise by practicing active relaxation for at least another ten minutes. After you perform both styles of progressive relaxation, you will probably be drawn to either active or passive. One probably will seem to work better or to mesh better with your personal style.

Feel free to choose whichever technique feels more comfortable and effective to complete every day, then use that one for the remainder of the program. While it probably won't hurt you to bounce back and forth between passive and active relaxation in the long run, I want you to get very comfortable with the technique that works best for you in order to get the most out of the program.

Remember, as you practice today, you probably won't feel

totally relaxed even after spending close to thirty minutes engaging in progressive relaxation. That's OK, because you are just learning how to use these techniques. Just do your best and understand that your ability to produce the relaxation response in your body using either relaxation technique will get only better and better. Now, go relax.

Assignment

- Practice passive relaxation for twenty minutes using CD Two or the guide at the end of today's reading.
- Practice active relaxation for ten to twenty minutes.

A GUIDE FOR PASSIVE RELAXATION

Get as comfortable as you possibly can. Sit back in a chair, or even lie down on a couch or a bed, and close your eyes. Take several deep breaths, making sure you breathe from the deepest part of your stomach and not your chest. Make sure your breaths are nice and slow. Inhale for the count of three, hold the breath, then exhale for the count of three. Repeat this several times.

As you take deep breaths in and out, imagine yourself on a lonely beach somewhere. Focus your attention on your hands. Imagine the bright, summer sun reflecting down on your hands, and feel the heat of the sun on your hands. As you continue to take deep breaths in and out, let your hands feel soft and relaxed. Say quietly to yourself in your head, "My hands are warm. They're soft. They're relaxed. They're pliable. My hands are extremely heavy." As you continue to breathe deeply, I want you to focus all your attention on your hands and let your hands feel heavy.

Now, shift your attention from your hands to your forearms as you continue to take deep breaths from your abdomen. As you sit on that beach, I want you to imagine the bright, summer sun reflecting on your forearms. And I want you to feel the warmth of the sun on your forearms. As you continue to take deep breaths in and out, let your forearms feel relaxed and soft. Say quietly to yourself, "My forearms are warm and soft; they're relaxed and pliable. My forearms feel extremely heavy." As you continue to breathe deeply, I want you to let your forearms feel heavy. Focus all your attention on your forearms. Feel the sun; feel the heat; feel the relaxation; feel the heaviness.

Keep breathing deeply now and shift your focus from your forearms to your biceps. Focus all your attention on your biceps. As you sit on that beach, imagine the bright summer sun reflecting down on your biceps, and feel the warmth of the sun on your biceps. Allow yourself to experience that heat. Let your biceps feel relaxed and soft. Say quietly, "My biceps are warm; they're soft; they're relaxed; they're pliable. My biceps are extremely heavy."

As you continue to breathe deeply, let your arms feel heavy—your hands, your forearms, your biceps. Let them feel heavy, and experience the warmth of the sun on your arms.

We're going to move now to your forehead. Focus all your attention on your forehead. This is where many people hold their stress. Recognize whether you have any stress in your forehead. I want you to begin to focus on all the stress in your forehead and allow that stress to just be drained out. Remember, you're sitting on that beach, and I want you to imagine the warm summer sun beating down on your forehead. You can feel it hitting your forehead. I want you to feel the warmth of that sun as the stress fades away from your forehead.

As you continue to take deep breaths in and out, I want you to let your forehead feel soft and relaxed. I want you to say quietly in your own head, "My forehead feels warm from the sun. It feels soft. It feels very relaxed." As you continue to breathe deeply, let your forehead feel extremely relaxed. And don't forget to breathe in and out.

Now continue that deep breathing as you shift focus from just your forehead to your entire face. As you continue to take deep breaths, I want you to move all your attention to your face. As you sit on that beach, I want you imagine the bright, summer sun reflecting down on your entire face. It's warm. You can feel the sun. As you continue to take deep breaths in and out, I want you to let your face feel extremely relaxed, soft, and pliable. Allow the stress to fade from your face. And I want you to tell yourself quietly, "My entire face feels warm; it feels soft; it feels relaxed."

And as you let that relaxation just resonate in your face, I want you to begin to shift focus. Breathe deeply as

37

you begin to concentrate on your shoulders. Tell yourself in your head, "My shoulders are beginning to feel soft. They're beginning to feel extremely relaxed." Remember, as you sit on that beach, I want you to imagine the bright sun reflecting down on your shoulders. It's hot. Feel the heat of the sun on your shoulders.

As you continue to breathe in and out, I want you to let your shoulders feel relaxed and soft. I want you to say quietly in your head, "My shoulders are incredibly warm; they're soft. My shoulders are relaxed. They feel pliable. My shoulders feel heavy." As you continue to breathe deeply from your stomach, let your shoulders feel heavy. Let them droop down. You can feel the warmth. You can feel the relaxation. And your shoulders feel heavy.

Now, I want you to focus your attention more on your stomach. Continue to breathe deeply as you focus on your entire abdomen. You're breathing deeply. Take a long breath from your stomach at the count of three, hold it, then let it go. As you sit on that beach, imagine the bright summer sun reflecting down on your abdomen. Continue to take deep breaths in and out, and let your stomach feel relaxed and soft. Tell yourself, "My stomach, my entire abdomen, feels soft and relaxed. My whole stomach feels heavy. My whole midsection is completely relaxed."

Now I want you to scan your entire upper body—your arms, your face, your shoulders, and your stomach. As you take deep breaths in and out, let your entire upper body feel soft, warm, and relaxed. Focus on any residual stress you have in your upper body, and let it go. Imagine that stress flowing up your upper body, down your arms, and out your fingertips. Let your whole upper body feel soft, warm, relaxed, and heavy.

Now we're going to shift focus. I want you to go from your upper body to your hamstrings. This is the top part of your legs. As you continue to breathe deeply, focus all your attention on your hamstrings. Imagine you're sitting on that beach, and you can feel the sunlight beaming down on your upper legs. It feels warm, and the heat of the sun is just beaming down. As you continue to take deep breaths in and out, your hamstrings feel soft and relaxed. I want you to say quietly to yourself, "My hamstrings feel so soft and relaxed. They feel warm from the sun. My hamstrings are incredibly heavy." As you take deep breaths in and out, let those hamstrings feel heavy. Take another deep breath.

Now shift your focus to your calves and feet. As you continue to breathe deeply, focus all your attention on your calves and feet. Remember, you're sitting on that beach, and that bright summer sun is reflecting down on your calves and feet.

You feel the warmth of the sun. You're taking deep breaths in and out. I want you to let your calves and feet feel relaxed and soft. I want you to say quietly, "My legs feel warm and soft. They're relaxed. They're pliable. My legs feel extremely heavy." As you continue to breathe deeply, I want you to let your entire lower body— everything below your waist—feel heavy.

Now scan your entire body for any signs of residual tension. Go from your hands to your arms to your face, your shoulders, your abdomen, your hamstrings, your calves, and your feet. Look for any signs of residual tension. As you breathe in and out slowly, the muscles in your hands and arms should feel very relaxed and very warm. Your hands should feel heavy. Say to yourself, "My hands feel extremely heavy." The muscles in your forearms should feel soft and pliable. Your forearms should feel heavy.

Now say to yourself in your head, "My forearms are relaxed." The muscles in your biceps should be smooth and loose. Say, "My biceps and my arms are extremely relaxed." The muscles in your forehead and your face should be relaxed and warm. Tell yourself, "My forehead and my face, they're loose. They're entirely relaxed." Remember, you're taking deep breaths in and out. As you take deep breaths in and out, notice that the muscles in your shoulders are very soft and pliable. Let your shoulders feel extremely heavy and loose. Say, "My shoulders are extremely heavy. They're relaxed."

The muscles in your stomach should be calm and relaxed. Let your stomach rise and fall rhythmically. Say, "My stomach muscles are extremely relaxed." The muscles in your hamstrings and upper legs should feel loose and smooth. Let both legs feel extremely heavy and say, "My legs are heavy." The muscles in your calves should feel soft and pliable. The muscles in your feet should feel incredibly loose and soft. Let your calf muscles and your feet feel extremely heavy and released. Say, "My feet, calves, and hamstrings feel extremely relaxed."

Now I want you to take another deep breath from your abdomen. Hold it for the count of three. As you exhale this time, allow any residual tension to drain away, allowing your entire body to relax very deeply all over. Again, take a deep breath and hold it. And again as you exhale, allow any residual tension left in your body to drain away. Allow your body to relax even deeper than before. As you continue to breathe in and out, let your entire body feel heavy. As you take some more deep breaths, say, "I am," as you inhale and, "relaxed," as you exhale. "I am. Relaxed." Practice that several times. Now take three more deep breaths. The third time open your eyes as you inhale. Then exhale, and take several more deep breaths.

Day Five

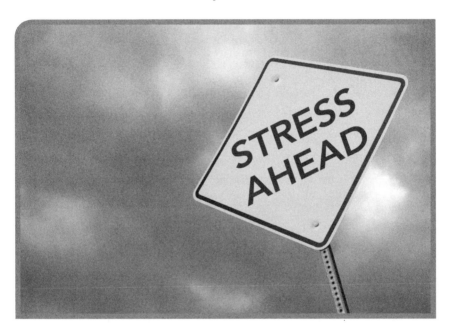

DISSECT YOUR STRESS

PRETEND WITH ME for a moment, OK? Imagine that everyone who lives with you has gone out of town for the weekend. It's Saturday night, and you have just spent the whole evening watching movies and eating popcorn. You go to bed exhausted and plan to sleep uninterrupted until at least 9:00 a.m. You fall asleep like a little baby and are catching some major REM sleep until...you wake up to the sound of a lamp crashing to the floor in the living room. What goes through your mind as you spring straight up and sit wide-awake in bed?

What would you tell yourself in this situation?

_____

_____

_____

When I propose this story to my counseling clients, most say the first thing that would run through their minds is something

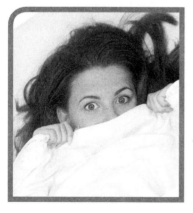

along these lines: "Oh, my gosh. There is someone in this house!" When I ask how they would feel in this situation, most clients say they would be scared or, to use a sophisticated, clinical term, *freaked-out*. When I ask what they would do, most mention something about finding a weapon to protect themselves or calling 911. (Occasionally, I get the brave client who assures me that he would run like a wild man into the living room determined to "pull a Rambo" on any would-be intruder.)

This illustration summarizes the typical response my clients give to this situation.

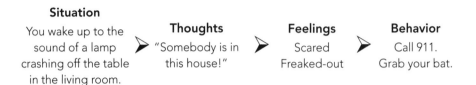

Situation
You wake up to the sound of a lamp crashing off the table in the living room.

Thoughts
"Somebody is in this house!"

Feelings
Scared
Freaked-out

Behavior
Call 911.
Grab your bat.

Now we are going to take this same scenario and change your perspective a little bit. You are still home alone at 3:00 a.m., and you still wake up to the sound of a lamp crashing off an end table in the living room. But let's say you have a new puppy, Sir Winston, in the house. Sir Winston is a wild dog, and he's been jumping up on that end table in the living room for days now. In fact, you've had to stop that lamp from falling off the table a hundred times. Now what goes through your mind?

What would you tell yourself in this situation now that Sir Winston is in the picture?

_____

_____

_____

When I confront my clients with the Sir Winston contingency, many say their thoughts would be dramatically different. Now they say they might tell themselves something like this: "That crazy dog. I should introduce him to the neighbor's doghouse." When asked what they would be feeling when this thought goes through their minds, they usually say they would be annoyed or irritated. When asked what they would do in this situation, most say they would roll over and go back to bed. The following illustration summarizes my clients' typical response in both scenarios.

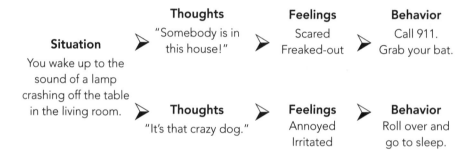

It's interesting, isn't it? The situation didn't change: in both instances you wake up to the sound of a lamp crashing off the table. But the way you think about the situation drastically affects the way you feel and what you do. When you think somebody is in the house, you feel scared, and that feeling drives your behavior. You call 911 or perhaps run into the living room in a Rambo-like fit of rage. But when you think the crazy dog knocked the lamp off the table, you feel annoyed, and that feeling drives your behavior. You roll over and go back to sleep.

You may find this little illustration amusing, but it demonstrates a powerful concept that is essential to your ability to manage stress: thoughts lead to feelings, and feelings lead to behavior. No matter what situation, environment, or relationship you encounter in life, the way you think about it will drive your feelings, and your feelings will drive your behavior.

If you think back to the reading from Day One, you'll understand why this concept is so key for living a less-stressed life. Remember, stress is the body's response to situations that we perceive and interpret as dangerous, overwhelming, or "impossible." The key words here are *perceive* and *interpret.* Just like in the scenario of the lamp crashing to the floor in the middle of the night, the thoughts you have about a situation will determine whether or not it is perceived as stressful. Stress is really all about the perspective you take on a situation; it is created by what you tell yourself the situation means.

Let me give you another example of how your thoughts help create and sustain your stress. Your boss walks into your office and says, "You're fired!" Is this situation stressful? Well, it depends on how you think about what just happened. Suppose you think something like this: "Oh, my. What am I going to do? I love this job, and I need the money so badly."

That thought will lead to some pretty stressed and anxious feelings. And those emotions probably will lead to some directed behavior, perhaps going to the Internet to look for new positions, running to your boss's office to grovel at his feet, or immediately filling your briefcase with as many office supplies as possible.

I know what some of you might be thinking, "This situation is inherently stressful. Regardless of how you think about it, getting fired is stressful." I would agree with that belief for the most part, but not entirely. Let's change the thoughts associated with this situation. Your boss still walks in and says you are fired. But let's say this time you sit down at your desk and say to yourself, "God must have something else in store for me. I know He'll see me and my family through this. Thankfully, I can draw unemployment while He leads me to another job that I enjoy." You're feeling significantly less stressed with these thoughts, aren't you? You might even feel a sense of anticipation. Your behavior might be drastically different as well. Rather than running to your boss's office to beg for your job back, you might start thinking of some of the things you'd always wanted to do but lacked time for because of your demanding job.

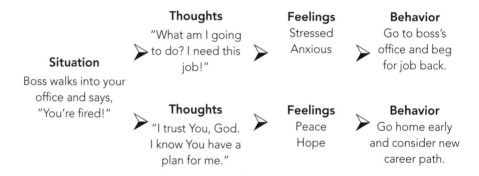

The most important thing to take from this example is to understand that your thoughts lead to your feelings, and your feelings lead to your behavior. Still not convinced? Let's consider another example. Your eight-year-old daughter asks to go to McDonald's for lunch. You kindly explain that she has eaten at McDonald's five times in the last forty-eight hours, and she needs to eat a healthier lunch. At that point her eight-year-old brain takes over, and she starts a long tirade that ends with, "I hate you!" What are you thinking?

Well, you have at least two options. You may think, "I can't believe she said that. I'm such a horrible parent. I can never make her happy." If you engage in that line of thinking, you're liable to feel inadequate, guilty, and stressed. Who knows what behavior these feelings will provoke? Maybe you will end up taking her to McDonald's, or perhaps you will hit the steering wheel.

Your other option in this situation is to take a different perspective. You could think, "You know, kids will be kids. She's just going to have to learn how to handle this kind of frustration." These thoughts are likely to cause less stressful feelings and may even produce determination and assurance instead. And your behavior? You'll probably just keep driving and go eat at a place you feel is appropriate.

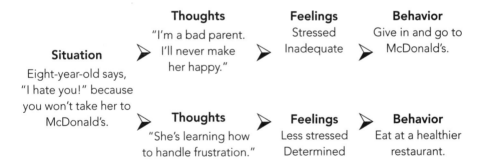

Are you starting to see the correlation among thoughts, feelings, and behavior a bit more clearly? Again, in this situation, your feeling of stress is not a result of the situation. It is a result of the way you *interpret* or *think about* the situation you are in.

One more example just to convince any naysayers out there: let's say your pastor spontaneously asks you to pray during one 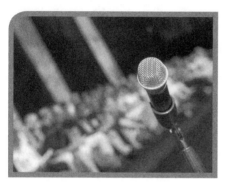 of the Sunday morning church services. You could think, "I can't believe he would do this. I haven't prepared for this at all. I'm going to sound like an idiot up there." If you respond this way, your feelings are likely to be at the high end of the stress spectrum. To use a very clinical term to describe this experience, you'd freak out.

Your behavior might be to slip out the back door during the morning announcements. Or you might decide to go ahead and pray, but to do so in a hesitant manner, complete with a cracked voice and timid posture. Another alternative would be to think differently about the situation, something along the lines of, "What an honor to be asked to pray during the service today. I am thrilled to be able to lead the congregation in worship. I'm not prepared, but I'll just speak from my heart." This train of thought will most definitely lead to less-stressed emotions—perhaps a settled feeling or maybe even confidence. Your behavior would likely be to step up to the stage confidently and to pray loudly and boldly.

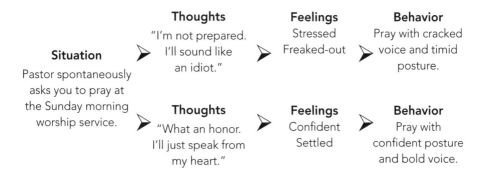

I hope you are getting it now. Thoughts lead to feelings, and feelings lead to behavior. In fact, your thoughts support and sustain your feelings just as scaffolding supports and sustains a building under construction. If you remove the scaffolding, the building will collapse. If you remove the thoughts that support your feelings, your feelings will collapse. So our stress is in us, not "out there." Our stress is not caused by our situation; it is caused by the way we think about the situations we find ourselves in. In any given circumstance, relationship, or environment we perceive as stressful, our thoughts drive and maintain our stress.

I hope you don't hear me saying that stress management is simple. It's not, and there are certain situations that clearly lend themselves to stress-inducing thoughts. That's why I had you complete the stress assessment. However, many chronically stressed people tend to have stress-inducing thoughts about a variety of situations, relationships, and environments. In short, when stress becomes a lifestyle, you can bet that they have laid down a pattern of engaging stress-inducing thoughts in multiple areas of their lives. This program is going to help you break that unhealthy pattern and learn how to live a less-stressed life.

49

The point of today's session is to highlight the relationship among your thoughts, feelings, and behavior. Tomorrow you will spend most of the time learning how to change your thoughts in the moment in order to live a less-stressed life. For now, I want you to concentrate on understanding your own stress-inducing thoughts, feelings, and behavior by listing your top five stress triggers.

Assignment

- Complete the Top Five Stress Triggers log.
- Practice passive or active relaxation for ten to twenty minutes.

TOP FIVE STRESS TRIGGERS

This log will help you tease out the kinds of situations you typically perceive as stressful and will highlight the degree to which your thoughts actually support and sustain your stress. Start your log by listing the top five stress-inducing situations you encounter on a consistent basis, with one being the most stressful and five the least stressful. Then try to piece together your thoughts, feelings, and behavior in these situations. If you are unsure about your thoughts, feelings, or behavior in a given situation, do your best to fill in that information the next time you encounter that particular circumstance, environment, or relationship.

Situation ➤	Thoughts ➤	Feelings ➤	Behaviors
1.			
2.			
3.			
4.			
5.			

Day Six

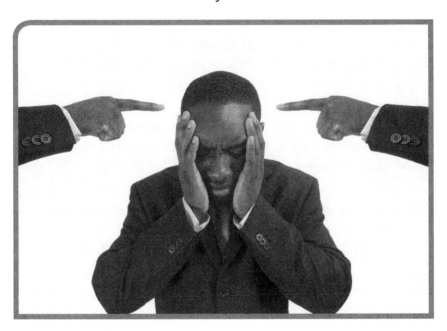

CLUE IN TO YOUR THOUGHTS AND FEELINGS

Have you started to make the connections between your stress-inducing thoughts, your feelings, and your behavior? I hope listing your top five stress triggers helped you do just that. Now you are ready to begin thinking about how to change your thoughts in the moment so that you can feel less stressed in any given situation, environment, or relationship. The key here is to become keenly aware of your thoughts on a moment-by-moment basis when you are in situations that trigger stress. When you are fully aware of your thoughts, you can begin to adjust them accordingly.

The problem is that it's impossible to be aware of all the thoughts that run through your head every second of every day. Think about it. We talk to ourselves internally more than we talk to anyone else. It's OK to admit that. I'm talking to myself in my head right now. I'm very hungry and can't wait to go get something to eat, but I won't get up out of this chair without thinking it through in my head.

When I finish this paragraph, I'll tell myself, "Well, let's go get something to eat. Maybe I'll try the Chinese place again. The last time was horrible, but, hey, everybody loses a hair while he is cooking now and then." This inner dialogue will happen all day as I engage many different environments.

It is impossible to monitor our thoughts twenty-four hours a day, seven days a week to catch any stress-inducing thoughts we may have. We just talk to ourselves too often. We have too many thoughts about ourselves, our lives, and the environments we encounter. In order to live a less-stressed life, we need to clue in to our thoughts, but we need to be selective about when we do this. It's important that we become aware of our thoughts when we first begin to experience some sort of internal feeling of stress.

If you pay close attention to your feeling of stress, you will have a chance to recognize the thoughts driving your emotions and change your perspective. This may seem like an easy thing to do, but most people don't recognize their feelings of stress in a given situation or environment until they are well into the process of stressing out. They ignore the subtle clues, and by the time they realize that they are indeed stressed, it's too late. They are completely overcome with the physical, emotional, or mental effects of stress.

Sound familiar? If you're like most people dealing with chronic stress, you probably don't realize you are stressing out until the headache hits, your stomach is tied in knots, your mind is racing so fast you can't keep up, or you just feel like an emotional wreck. And if you wait until then to begin to manage your stress, you will surely fail. At that point you are too caught up in the physical, emotional, mental, relational, or spiritual effects of your stress to take appropriate action.

It's human nature. When your stress feels out of control, your main goal is simply to survive the situation, not necessarily to correct the underlying problem. If you want to live a less-stressed life, it is vitally important that you become keenly aware of your emotions so you can recognize the early signs of stress manifesting in your life.

The only way to become more emotionally aware is to practice. I know this may sound odd, but you can become a student of your emotions in general and your stress levels in particular. You can study your emotional experience on a consistent basis to tease out when feelings of stress are very subtly starting to stir within you. When you can catch yourself on the front end of stress, you are in a good position to begin cluing in to the thoughts that are driving it.

Focus on Your Stress-Inducing Thoughts

You will find a stress log at the end of today's reading that will help you practice becoming more aware of when your stress starts emotionally. As you become more aware of your thoughts, you will probably begin to see themes or categories emerge that are without question stress inducing. Researchers have identified several different kinds of thoughts that typically lead to stress. I call these "hot thoughts," meaning they will usually lead to a significant experience of stress. I've included a summary of some of these thoughts so you can identify any that are at work in your life.[1]

- All-or-Nothing Thoughts. Individuals with these hot thoughts tend to see things in absolute, black-and-white categories. Example: "Either I am perfectly competent in everything I do, or I am a failure."

- Overgeneralization. People with these thoughts assume bad events will happen over and over, or that things are always a certain way. Example: "The neighborhood dogs will always choose to relieve themselves on my lawn."

- Mental Filter. This type of hot thought causes a person to focus on the negative parts of life and filter out the positive. Example: "My job is awful because I don't get paid enough." (But he will

overlook the fact that he has good work condi-
tions, hours, etc.)

- Magnification and Globalization. People with
  these hot thoughts magnify their mistakes and
  make them a big deal. Example: "I'm terrible with
  the kids because I just yelled at them."

- Personalization. These hot thoughts lead a person
  to accept blame for negative events involving
  others. Example: "My family would be well
  adjusted if it weren't for me."

Although not all your hot thoughts will fall neatly into these
categories, you will probably see some themes that are consistent with one or more of these tendencies. As you begin to clue
in to your thoughts on a consistent basis, take note of which
category (or categories) seems to best reflect your thought life.

Tomorrow we will talk about what to do with these kinds of
hot thoughts when you are able to identify them in the moment.
In the meantime, it's important that you practice cluing in to
your thoughts when you begin to feel stress. You can't monitor
your thoughts all day every day, but you can use the feeling of
stress as a signal to focus in on the thoughts you are having
about yourself, a particular situation, or other people.

Trust me, this is harder than it seems because the more
intense a situation becomes emotionally, the more difficult it
is to find the energy to attend to your thoughts. Don't get me
wrong: cluing in to your thoughts when you're feeling stressed
is not impossible, but you must intentionally practice these
skills.

This is why I created the stress log. This form will help you practice cluing in to your thoughts and feelings on the front end of a stressful experience. This is critically important, so I am going to ask you to complete this form every day for the rest of the program. Because the skill of recognizing your thoughts and feelings during stressful times is obviously of the utmost importance, please take this portion of the program seriously.

The stress log will help you pay close attention to your internal experience by encouraging you to intentionally log your thoughts and feelings every few hours throughout the day, regardless of whether or not you are feeling stressed. Honestly, the program becomes quite demanding at this point. It is hard to remember to carry a stress log with you all day and to fill it out every so often. But keep in mind that your future won't change until you intentionally change the present.

On the first day you begin filling out your stress log (which I hope is Day Six of the program for you), you need only to log the first four columns. By the end of your reading on Day Seven, you will know how to complete every column of the stress log and will be well on your way to challenging the thoughts that are creating and supporting your stress.

Assignment

- Complete the first four columns of the stress log.
- Practice passive or active relaxation for twenty minutes.

STRESS LOG

This stress log will help you practice becoming more aware of the emotions you experience when your stress begins. On Day Six, complete only the first four columns.

	Situation	Thought	Feeling	Behavior	NEW Thought	NEW Feeling	NEW Behavior
Breakfast to Lunch							
Lunch to Dinner							
Dinner to Bedtime							

Day Seven

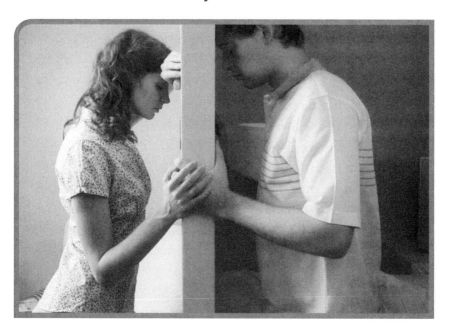

CHALLENGE YOUR
STRESS-INDUCING THOUGHTS

I HOPE YOU HAVE had some success logging your thoughts and feelings. Remember, your journey to a less-stressed life is just starting, and much of what you are discovering has a fairly steep learning curve. Expect that it will be difficult to clue in to your thoughts and feelings initially, but if you stick with it, you will become much more aware of your internal experience. My hunch is that you will be surprised by how negative and stress-inducing your thoughts actually are.

At this point you're probably wondering, "What now? Now that I am becoming more aware of how my thoughts are causing the stress response in my body, what do I do about it?" Good question. When you identify a stress-inducing thought soon after encountering a stressful situation, you are in a great position to challenge the thought and then change it.

Let's look at an example that will illustrate how to do this. Let's say you are talking with your spouse about politics. You are a staunch Republican, and your spouse has been "leaning left" since you were married. Although you may not have talked much about politics while you were dating, it has been a point of contention for some time now. During this conversation you try to convey the importance of voting for the Republican candidate for city council.

Although your spouse has listened to your arguments intently, he or she is still convinced the best choice is the Independent candidate. About five minutes into the conversation, you realize your heart rate is up, you are sweating more than usual, and you are feeling quite stressed by your spouse's inability to see your point of view. Your thoughts are centered on how "ridiculous" your spouse's views are and on how difficult it is to communicate with someone so closed-minded.

Your behavior is increasingly hostile and aggressive. I've summarized what we know so far about your stress process in this stress log.

Situation					
My spouse does not agree with me about the merits of the Republican candidate for city council.					
Thought	**Feeling**	**Behavior**	**NEW Thought**	**NEW Feeling**	**NEW Behavior**
"I can't believe the person I love is being so ridiculous."	Stressed	Raised voice			
"There is just no getting this person to listen to good, logical reasoning."	Frustrated	Aggressive posture			

With this information about your internal experience, you are in a position to begin challenging the thoughts that are producing your stress. In order to do this, you need to ask yourself a simple question: "Is there another way to look at this situation?" This one question can have a tremendous impact upon your stress level almost immediately because it opens you up to other possible perspectives on the situation. Basically, by asking this question you are communicating to yourself, in no uncertain terms, that the stress-producing thought is not working very well for you. It might be a valid perspective, but if it is creating stress, that line of thinking must go.

It's important to note that I am not asking you to consider unrealistic ways to think about the situation, but to consider other, equally valid ways to understand what is happening to you at that moment. Let's go back to our example and practice a little bit. Is there another way to think about a spouse who is not open to your arguments about the Republican candidate for city council?

What could you tell yourself in this situation that would be less stress inducing?

_____

_____

_____

_____

Rather than "ridiculous," perhaps another way to define your spouse's behavior is "passionate." Maybe another way to think about your spouse's "closed-mindedness" is to define that trait as "principled." And did your spouse really refuse to listen to you, or did he or she listen objectively and then form an independent conclusion? How are you going to feel if you choose to believe the equally valid view that your spouse is passionate and principled rather than ridiculous and closed-minded? Without a doubt you will feel less stressed. Let's look at the stress log to see how the new thoughts will affect your feelings and behavior.

Situation					
My spouse does not agree with me about the merits of the Republican candidate for city council.					
Thought	**Feeling**	**Behavior**	**NEW Thought**	**NEW Feeling**	**NEW Behavior**
"I can't believe the person I love is being so ridiculous."	Stressed	Raised voice	"I am blessed to have such a passionate individual in my life."	Less stressed	Listening respectfully
"There is just no getting this person to listen to good, logical reasoning."	Frustrated	Aggressive posture	"It is nice to see the one I love standing firm on principle. I might not agree, but I respect the integrity I see here."	Proud	Open body language

I know this entire process might seem like a stretch to you because everyone knows how challenging it is to change a long-standing pattern, especially a long-standing thought pattern. However, it is possible. You will find that as you begin to argue with yourself and challenge your stress-inducing thoughts, you will truly feel less stressed. It's a difficult process, no doubt, but it is extremely effective.

You are now ready to begin filling out your stress log completely. As stressful situations arise, start diffusing them by taking the time to assess your thoughts, feelings, and behavior, and then to write them down. Then begin to ask yourself the important question, "Is there another way to look at this situation?" Don't be afraid to be creative and write down any other thoughts that might produce less stress. Think about the feelings and behavior that will emerge if you can let the new thoughts saturate your mind, then write them down.

Although there is no guarantee that you will be able to quickly adjust your thinking in the middle of your stress process, at least you'll be paying attention to your internal experience. For the next few days you will be exposed to even more information about the source of your stress-producing thoughts. Armed with this new information, you will be able to "switch gears" more readily.

Because the stress log is obviously one of the foundations of this program, I want you to focus on filling it out every day for the rest of this program. Continue to log your thoughts and feelings at least three times a day, no matter what. Even as you see the program working and you begin to feel less stressed, keep logging your thoughts and feelings.

In addition to the three built-in log entries (between breakfast and lunch, lunch and dinner, and dinner and bedtime), complete all seven columns of the stress log every time you notice that you are *starting* to feel stressed. Again, you might not be able to break out of your stress immediately, but you will be growing more aware of the connection between your thoughts, feelings, and behavior.

Assignment

- Practice passive or active relaxation for twenty minutes.
- Log thoughts, feelings, and behavior three times a day after breakfast, after lunch, and before bedtime using the stress log.
- Complete all seven columns of the stress log when you *begin* to feel stressed.

STRESS LOG

This stress log will help you practice becoming more aware of the emotions you experience when your stress begins. It should be completed daily beginning on Day Six of the Stress Relief for Life program. If you encounter a stressful experience during your day, fill out the entire row under the appropriate time period. If you don't have a stressful experience, complete only the first four columns.

	Situation	Thought	Feeling	Behavior	NEW Thought	NEW Feeling	NEW Behavior
Breakfast to Lunch							
Lunch to Dinner							
Dinner to Bedtime							

Day Eight

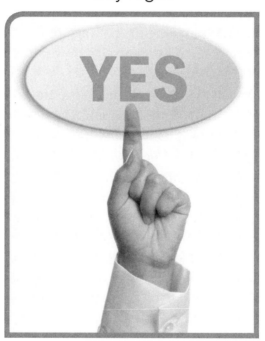

GET TO THE CORE OF YOUR STRESS: PEOPLE PLEASING

S O ARE YOU convinced that your stress is created by hot thoughts that lead to the feeling of stress? My guess is that you are surprised by how stress inducing your thoughts actually are. That's a good thing because having insight into your stress process is half the battle—which leads us to our topic for today. Now that you are cluing in to your hot thoughts and beginning to challenge those thoughts, you are probably starting to ask yourself, "How in the world did I ever start thinking this way?"

Good question. The answer is related to the brokenness we discussed at the start of the program. Our lives really aren't supposed to be this way. Our minds aren't supposed to be saturated with the kinds of negative and fearful thoughts that drive stress. God never intended this. But because of the state of our world and the relationships we engage in, we are faced with a tremendous amount of brokenness early in our lives. In fact, we usually learn core beliefs about ourselves, about how the world works, and about how to be in a relationship with others from our families and our early experiences with peers.

Think about it. Where did you learn how to maintain connectedness with other people? When did you adopt the beliefs you have about what makes you significant? Where did you learn how to gain acceptance and avoid isolation? You learned these core beliefs early in life from your parents, your siblings, and your interaction with kids at school or in the neighborhood.

These core beliefs about ourselves, the world, and others are the foundation upon which we build our thoughts in any given situation, relationship, or environment. In other words, the hot thoughts that drive our stress were developed within the context of the core beliefs about life we learned in childhood.

Allow me to explain the connection between our hot thoughts and these core beliefs in more detail. Remember the scenario we discussed earlier about the eight-year-old who wanted to go to McDonald's?

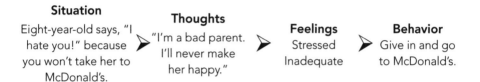

Situation	Thoughts	Feelings	Behavior
Eight-year-old says, "I hate you!" because you won't take her to McDonald's.	"I'm a bad parent. I'll never make her happy."	Stressed Inadequate	Give in and go to McDonald's.

In this situation you experienced a dramatic hot thought that was clearly a globalization of the situation. Where did this idea come from? People who have these kinds of thoughts often have a people-pleasing core belief driving or creating their hot thoughts.

The people-pleasing core belief tells you that you are acceptable, worthwhile, significant, lovable, or "OK" if other people approve of you and your actions. The opposite is true as well: the people-pleasing core belief also tells you that you are not acceptable, worthwhile, significant, or lovable—you're just not OK—if other people don't approve of you and your actions.

In the situation with the eight-year-old, you could have responded in any number of ways to the child's reply of "I hate you." Why would anyone automatically think he is a bad person? Probably because somewhere down deep inside, the individual believed that his worth as a parent was based on whether or not his children liked, appreciated, and affirmed him. A summary of this stress process would probably look something like this.

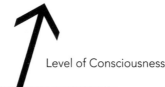

Situation	Thoughts	Feelings	Behavior
Eight-year-old says, "I hate you!" because you won't take her to McDonald's.	"I'm a bad parent. I'll never make her happy."	Stressed Inadequate	Give in and go to McDonald's.

Level of Consciousness

Core Beliefs
People Pleasing
"If other people approve of me, I'm OK. If other people don't approve of me, I'm not OK."

"If my children like me, I'm a good parent, but if they don't like me, then I'm a bad parent."

"If I make other people happy, then I'm successful and good at relationships. If I make people unhappy, I'm a miserable failure at relationships."

The Difference Between Core Beliefs and Hot Thoughts

Although hot thoughts are driven by core beliefs, there are some important distinctions. The most important distinction is their source. Hot thoughts are responses to specific situations. In contrast, core beliefs are general rules about life learned early on that cut across many situations. Let's say a guy named

Jim who is having his new girlfriend over for dinner burns the steak to a charred black crisp. He gets really stressed-out and eventually just orders takeout in tears. (His girlfriend ends up leaving early because, well, out-of-control emotions have a way of making dinner pretty uncomfortable.)

In his most stressful moment, Jim tells himself, "I'm such a bad cook; everything I do fails." This hot thought was a direct response to the steaks. His underlying core belief—"I must be competent in everything I do to be a good person"—is more general. This core belief fuels his hot thoughts when he burns steak, when he arrives late for work, when he forgets his paperwork for a staff meeting, and every other time he makes a mistake.

I know what you're thinking: "I've never even thought about this whole concept of core beliefs, and I sure don't remember thinking anything like, 'If other people don't like me or approve of me, then I'm not OK.'" I know. That's the point. Typically you can't point to core beliefs consciously; they lie beneath your conscious awareness. But there is good news: although core beliefs aren't immediately conscious, you can figure out what your core beliefs are if you want to because they aren't totally unconscious either. They are actually what I call "preconscious," which means you can access your core beliefs if you take the time to analyze them.

Do You Have a People-Pleasing Core Belief?

Are you a good team player? Are you easy to get along with? Do you pride yourself on being laid-back and a master of avoiding conflict? If you answered yes to any of these questions, you might lean toward a people-pleasing core belief. In short, this belief system causes people to seek the approval of others in order to feel significant, worthwhile, lovable, and worthy of connection. Some examples of the thoughts that drive a people-pleasing core belief include:

- To be a good person, everyone must approve of the things I do.
- If people really knew me, they would think I am terrible, weak, and uninteresting.
- I am fully responsible for the feelings of others.
- Others will love me more if I am always selfless.
- People are bound to reject me.

Although your core beliefs might sound a little different from these examples, if you are a people pleaser, you will get stressed when others do not approve of you or your behavior. In order to determine if you have a people-pleasing core belief, look back over your recent stress logs. Do you see any themes in the hot thoughts that drive your stress? Do you see any patterns surfacing around people pleasing in particular? If you consistently have thoughts that center on stress over not pleasing others, being rejected, or being in conflict with others, you probably have a people-pleasing core belief.

Another way that you can figure out if people-pleasing issues are causing some of your hot thoughts is to think intentionally about your experience growing up. Think about your interaction with your mom and dad, brothers and sisters, and friends from the neighborhood or school. Obviously, most people will be more comfortable thinking about the more positive childhood memories. But as you consider the breadth of your experience as a child, and even as a teenager, do you have significant memories of feeling rejected, blamed, or teased? If so, you probably have some people-pleasing core beliefs that are driving some of your hot thoughts.

I know you may have questions about why I'm discussing core beliefs during a stress-relief program. You'll see during your reading on Day Eleven why core beliefs are so important for living a less-stressed life. For now, just know that the more you understand your core beliefs and how they drive your hot thoughts, the more power you will have over your stress.

In the meantime, I want you to continue to complete your stress log on a consistent basis and look for opportunities to challenge your hot thoughts in the moment. You should start to see some improvement in your ability to be insightful about how your thoughts are causing your stress. You might even find relief from some of your stress as you evaluate other equally valid ways to think about stress-inducing situations.

Assignment

- Practice passive or active relaxation for twenty minutes.
- Log thoughts, feelings, and behavior three times a day after breakfast, after lunch, and before bedtime using the stress log.
- Complete all seven columns of the stress log when you *begin* to feel stressed.

STRESS LOG

This stress log will help you practice becoming more aware of the emotions you experience when your stress begins. It should be completed daily beginning on Day Six of the Stress Relief for Life program. If you encounter a stressful experience during your day, fill out the entire row under the appropriate time period. If you don't have a stressful experience, complete only the first four columns.

	Situation	Thought	Feeling	Behavior	NEW Thought	NEW Feeling	NEW Behavior
Breakfast to Lunch							
Lunch to Dinner							
Dinner to Bedtime							

Day Nine

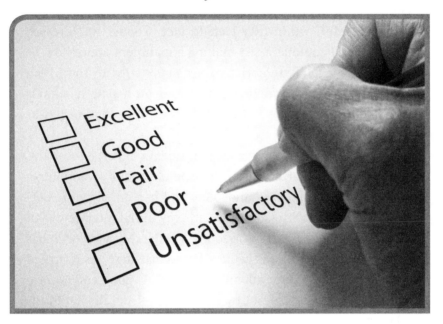

GET TO THE CORE OF YOUR STRESS: PERFORMANCE AND CONTROL

'LL NEVER FORGET the day Cooper walked into my counseling office. He was the picture of competence, intellect, and success. He was one of the most physically fit individuals I had seen in real life, and his imposing stature was accented with a fine-looking, obviously expensive Italian suit. He was dripping with so much jewelry that he could set off any metal detector within fifty feet. In fact, Cooper was dressed so well that I couldn't resist making a comment about how he brought back fond memories of my many trips to the Milan fashion shows. (Considering that I had on a pair of khakis and a Polo shirt, Cooper was well aware this statement was intended to be humorous.)

Cooper was the executive vice president of a large company, a position he had attained by the ripe old age of twenty-nine. He had a great job, was handsome, and had an engaging personality. As I sat with Cooper during my initial interview with him, I couldn't help but think to myself, "Here is a guy who has it all. Why in the world is he here for counseling?" As it turned out, Cooper did have it all, but it still wasn't good enough. He was extremely stressed-out by everything—from his job to his relationship with his wife to his vexing golf swing. In every area of his life, Cooper was stressed, and his stress was taking its toll physically, emotionally, and spiritually.

During his initial counseling sessions, I asked Cooper to complete exercises similar to the ones found in this program. He completed stress logs and eventually became more aware of his thoughts and feelings when he was in stressful situations. Over time, Cooper found that his stress was created and supported by thoughts like, "I'm never going to keep up with my work and still be the kind of husband I need to be." Other hot thoughts were: "I'd be a decent friend if I were more caring and available." "There is no way that I am ever going to amount to anything professionally."

An over-focus on his performance was the major theme of Cooper's hot thoughts, and this thought pattern cut across multiple situations and environments. Cooper was convinced at a deep level that he was only significant and worthy of love from others if he performed well all the time. The minute his performance as an employee, friend, or husband was less than perfect, Cooper got stressed—really stressed. Despite his tremendous success physically, professionally, relationally, and spiritually, he was stressed anytime he thought he had "missed the mark."

Cooper had a performance-based core belief. This core belief is rooted in the assumption that you obtain connection, love, significance, and worth because of your performance. People with performance-based core beliefs confuse *who they are* with *what they do.* They mistake lovability with performance. Here are some examples of the thoughts that undergird this core belief:

- If I'm competent all the time, people will respect me.
- Love must be earned with unusual accomplishments.
- If I can create a positive outcome, then I'm OK; if the outcome is not good, then I'm not OK.
- I should be productive all the time.

- Perfection is the only acceptable standard (at work, in relationships, in my Christian walk, etc.).
- If I look and sound intelligent, then I'll be respected and loved.

The performance-based core belief can be expressed in a person's life in a number of different ways. However, whenever someone with a performance-based core belief is convinced that he has not performed well, he will experience some form of stress. Remember our example of the pastor who spontaneously asked you to pray at the Sunday morning worship service? Here's the summary of how things went south when the hot thought led to stressful feelings:

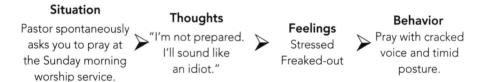

Situation
Pastor spontaneously asks you to pray at the Sunday morning worship service.

Thoughts
"I'm not prepared. I'll sound like an idiot."

Feelings
Stressed Freaked-out

Behavior
Pray with cracked voice and timid posture.

This is a classic example of a hot thought that was driven by a performance-based core belief. The hot thought ("I'm not prepared; I'll sound like an idiot") is clearly based on the general assumption that your worth and significance are directly related to your ability to produce a thoughtful prayer in the pulpit. In short, a performance-based core belief that said you could live with yourself only if you had a positive outcome was creating significant stress. I've summarized this stress process for you.

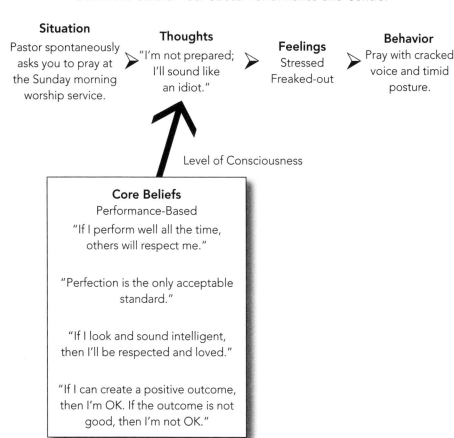

Situation
Pastor spontaneously asks you to pray at the Sunday morning worship service.

Thoughts
"I'm not prepared; I'll sound like an idiot."

Feelings
Stressed
Freaked-out

Behavior
Pray with cracked voice and timid posture.

Level of Consciousness

Core Beliefs
Performance-Based

"If I perform well all the time, others will respect me."

"Perfection is the only acceptable standard."

"If I look and sound intelligent, then I'll be respected and loved."

"If I can create a positive outcome, then I'm OK. If the outcome is not good, then I'm not OK."

Vying for Control?

Not many people who come to counseling bop into my office the way Denise did, so I was quite intrigued by our first meeting. To say that Denise exuded magnetic energy would be an understatement. She was light, breezy, and even quite funny as we went over the preliminary information from her paperwork. When I asked her directly why she was coming for counseling, Denise said bluntly, "I need someone to help me straighten out my husband. He is being unresponsive to my needs and the needs of my family." I was taken aback. How was she talking with such ease about such a painful experience? As I continued to listen during the initial session, I began to see a fuller picture.

For several years, Denise had controlled her family in general and her husband, Daryl, in particular. She made the decisions about how the kids were disciplined, where they went out to eat, how the money was spent, and what leisure activities the family pursued. After ten years, Daryl finally rebelled. First, he started enjoying some new hobbies on his own. Then he told Denise that he was through being her yes-man. Obviously, none of this sat well with Denise, and she started to experience serious symptoms of stress.

Although her stress was somewhat understandable considering the situation, I was amazed at her response to Daryl's new behavior. As her stress levels rose, she would attempt to control Daryl through more and more aggressive means. And the more hostile Denise was, the more convinced she became that Daryl was rebelling. Denise was so energized during our initial session because she was convinced I would agree that her stress was a direct result of her husband's rebellion.

I made the decision to work with Denise for several sessions to determine what in the world was going on with her controlling nature. Her hot thoughts centered on helplessness and powerlessness. When Daryl spent money without consulting her first, Denise told herself, "He is not even trying to respect my wishes when it comes to the finances." She reported that when Daryl would spend money without asking her, she often would immediately come down with stomachaches and headaches. Denise would experience these physiological responses even though they were very secure financially.

82

Daryl's newfound autonomy brought other struggles for Denise. When Daryl joined a tennis league, she experienced significant stress. Her hot thoughts again centered on helplessness and powerlessness: "I can't believe he is abandoning the family every Saturday morning like this. He won't even listen to logical reasoning about why he should be home for us on the weekend."

The issues between Denise and Daryl were complicated, but it became clear early in our sessions that one of the problems Denise was dealing with was a core belief that focused on controlling others. Denise's core belief told her, "Others must do what I think they should do, or they don't love me." This core belief was causing some hot thoughts that were generating a fairly stress-filled experience.

People with control-based core beliefs usually focus their efforts on controlling other people or on controlling themselves. People who focus on self-control are often not stressed if they maintain their discipline and predictability. But when they miss the mark and fail to follow through on their "schedule" or "routine," they really stress out. When an individual is invested in controlling others, he is often respected for his convictions but viewed as hard to get along with. Just like Denise, when others step out of line (i.e., they don't do what the controlling person thinks they should do), that usually provokes serious stress. Some examples of the thoughts underlying control-based core beliefs include:

- "If things don't go as I have planned, I am out of control, and that means something bad about me" (self-control).

- "If others don't do as I wish, they do not care about me or respect me" (control of others).

- "I must be strong because only the strong are valued, respected, and loved" (self-control and control of others).

- "If anything goes wrong, it is my fault" (control of others).

Let's look at the example we discussed previously about the political conversation with your spouse. Here's a summary of how your hot thoughts in the moment can lead to serious stress.

Situation
My spouse does not agree with me about the merits of the Republican candidate for city council.

Thoughts
"I can't believe the person I love is being so ridiculous."

Feelings
Stressed
Frustrated

Behavior
Raised voice
Aggressive posture

This example demonstrates how subtle the power of a control-based core belief can be. In the moment, the hot thought isn't even focused on control. However, using the word *ridiculous* suggests that you are uncomfortable when others disagree with you or when you can't control their opinion. The feeling of frustration also reflects a core belief rooted in control. Many times people who struggle with control-based core beliefs have an angry stress experience where the emotions of stress and anger are intermingled and indistinguishable from each other. A summary of this stress process follows.

Situation
My spouse does not agree with me about the merits of the Republican candidate for city council.

Thoughts
"I can't believe the person I love is being so ridiculous."

Feelings
Stressed
Frustrated

Behavior
Raised voice
Aggressive posture

Level of Consciousness

Core Beliefs
Control-Based
"If people agree with my opinion, that means they respect me."

"If conversations don't go my way, there is something bad about me or the other person."

"I must be 'right' in order to be worthwhile and significant."

What's Driving You?

Do you have any performance- or control-based beliefs? Do you get stressed when you can't control yourself or other people? Do you confuse your lovability with performance? If you're not sure, look at the stress logs you have completed so far. Consistent themes in hot thoughts point to specific core beliefs.

Have any patterns surfaced surrounding your performance? Do your hot thoughts consistently focus on pressure to "do more" at work or home? Do you find yourself stressing about whether or not you "look stupid" or have done something "right"? If so, you probably struggle with a performance-based core belief.

How about control? Do you consistently stress out over whether or not you follow through with your self-designed schedule? Do you experience stress when other people don't agree with you or comply with your requests? If so, you may be struggling with a control-based core belief.

Take some time today to think about what's beneath your hot thoughts. In particular, consider your experience growing up. Think about interactions with your parents, your friends from the neighborhood, and your siblings. Does anything stick out that seems consistent with an over-focus on performance or control? People with performance-based core beliefs often will have positive memories about their early life that center around achievement and success, and negative memories that are focused on inadequacy or the pressure to do more. Individuals with control-based core beliefs often will have negative memories of discipline or a lack of freedom, and positive memories of independence and freedom.

If you can't speak with any certainty about your core beliefs yet, don't worry. We'll pick up the whole idea of core beliefs again during tomorrow's reading.

Assignment

- Practice passive or active relaxation for twenty minutes.
- Log thoughts, feelings, and behavior three times a day after breakfast, after lunch, and before bedtime using the stress log.
- Complete all seven columns of the stress log when you *begin* to feel stressed.

STRESS LOG

This stress log will help you practice becoming more aware of the emotions you experience when your stress begins. It should be completed daily beginning on Day Six of the Stress Relief for Life program. If you encounter a stressful experience during your day, fill out the entire row under the appropriate time period. If you don't have a stressful experience, complete only the first four columns.

	Situation	Thought	Feeling	Behavior	NEW Thought	NEW Feeling	NEW Behavior
Breakfast to Lunch							
Lunch to Dinner							
Dinner to Bedtime							

Day Ten

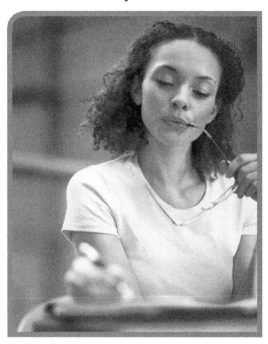

THE OLD STORY

A RE YOU STILL having a problem identifying the core beliefs beneath your stress? Don't worry. Sometimes it is tough to develop a sense of what is influencing our thoughts. It might take awhile for you to develop real insight into which core beliefs are operating in your life.

This process might be especially complicated if you truly struggle with more than one theme in your system of core beliefs. For instance, it is quite possible for you to identify situations where you struggle with people-pleasing *and* performance-based core beliefs. In other environments you might see yourself operating on a control-based core belief.

My purpose in introducing you to the whole concept of core beliefs is not to have you place yourself rigidly into one of these categories. Rather, it is to help you better understand what typically drives your stress in different environments. If you find that you are a people-pleaser in some situations and a control freak in others, that's great. Having a rich understanding of your core beliefs ultimately will help you get the most out of the Stress Relief for Life program.

Do you still need more help recognizing the core beliefs that are driving your hot thoughts? Examining your understanding of God will be helpful because we often project our core beliefs onto Him. Let me give you an example. Have you ever known a perfectionist, someone who probably had a very strong performance-based core belief? That was Gail. When she came in for her initial counseling appointment, it was clear early on that she had the tendency to work out her faith with an over-focus on her spiritual performance.

Although she had intellectual knowledge of the concept of grace, she was merciless with herself when it came to spiritual disciplines such as prayer, Bible study, worship, and medita-tion. She could believe God loved her if she spent an hour in prayer during the day, but she struggled to feel God's accep-tance if she spent only twenty minutes in prayer. Gail's view of God was a projection of her performance-based core belief because we know from Scripture that prayer connects us to God, but it doesn't make us acceptable to Him. Unfortunately, Gail's experience is not uncommon. If you want a rich under-standing of your core beliefs, pay close attention to your views about God and His acceptance and affirmation of you.

Completing the Progress Report From God might give you even more insight into your core beliefs. After you answer the questions, think about your ideas about God's acceptance and affirmation of you. Do you feel that God loves you if you are strong and in control of yourself? If so, you probably have a control-based core belief. Do you sense God's affirmation when you have performed well in some spiritual capacity? If this is the case, you might have a performance-based core belief. Do you believe God loves you more when you are pleasing others or meeting their needs? This might mean you have a people-pleasing core belief.

PROGRESS REPORT FROM GOD

Have you ever received a performance review from your employer? If God were writing a progress report about you, what would He say? Your answers will probably give you more clues into the content of your core beliefs. However, if this exercise is going to be helpful to you, it is important to answer the following questions honestly. Don't give responses that you think are "theologically correct" or "Christian." Focus in on your natural, gut reactions.

PERFORMANCE EVALUATION

From: God

To: [your name] _____

Your strengths as a person of faith are as follows:

_____

_____

_____

After reviewing your life, you need improvement in the following areas:

_____

_____

_____

I feel you are at your best when you:

_____

_____

_____

I am especially pleased with you when you:

_____

_____

What's Your Old Story?

I hope you are getting a better sense of the core beliefs that drive your hot thoughts. As you look back over your stress logs, your early experience in childhood and adolescence, and your view of God, you should start to see some themes. If you continue to think through your core beliefs over the next couple of days, you should be able to answer with more insight the question, What makes me acceptable, worthwhile, significant, worthy of connection, and lovable?

Your goal for the remainder of today's session is to customize your core beliefs. I want you to begin to put the abstract concept of core beliefs into the context of your life by understanding how your core beliefs really sound in your own head. The goal here is to understand how the issues of people pleasing, performance, and control play out in the details of your life. The easiest way to do this is to write a story—about you. It should be an autobiography about how people pleasing, performance, and control issues have caused stress in specific relationships, environments, and situations.

Writing a story about yourself is helpful because people learn better by listening to stories than by listening to facts. That's why I've been using stories to illustrate the concepts of the Stress Relief for Life program. I've included an exercise at the end of today's reading that will help you think through the different components of your old story. As you write, don't focus on grammar or syntax. It doesn't have to be a pretty story, just a short, narrative account in which you illustrate the power that your core beliefs have had over your stress process. Remember the immensely talented and competent businessman named Cooper I told you about previously? I've included an excerpt of the story he wrote as an example.

COOPER'S OLD STORY

My name is Cooper, and I live life pretty stressed. I have always been extremely concerned about my performance. I guess at my core I feel I'm a worthwhile and significant person if I do things well. If I ever face a situation in which I don't do something right or perfectly, I get really down on myself and don't feel very worthwhile. I'm not sure where I got this from (my dad was pretty hard on me, I guess). But I know that my concern about my performance and doing things "right" and "with excellence" stresses me out in many areas of my life.

My focus on how well I perform probably has caused the most problems in my marriage. I don't have any kids yet, but that's probably because I'm real concerned that I won't be a good enough dad. My wife gets frustrated with my perfectionism, and I sometimes end up majoring on the minors. For instance, my wife accuses me of stressing more about whether or not our lawn looks good than whether or not I am connecting with her.

Of course, my issues with performance cause significant stress at the office. I get so stressed-out when I feel like my reports to my boss are not perfect, and I end up spending an inordinate amount of time on them. I'm always under the gun with deadlines because I spend so much time trying to micromanage my team. I guess I try to hold everyone else up to my standard of perfection, and I get really stressed when no one delivers (even me).

Some people say I've done well professionally, but I feel like a fake. I don't really deserve the position I'm in, and I'm afraid that it's only a matter of time until everyone finds out.

Spiritually, I'm a mess. God and I do well when I feel like I am being a good person. But the whole grace thing just doesn't make sense. If I lose track of Bible study or miss an opportunity to share my faith, I feel like I've failed God, and it takes me several weeks to find the courage to go to God about it.

One other area that I get stressed about is my appearance. I am obsessed with my body, and I work out an average of two hours a day. I'm in decent shape, but I'm not really satisfied with my body. I get stressed because of my appearance, but also because I spend so much time trying to get the body I feel like I'll never have.

Summary: My worth and my ability to feel loved by God and others are based on whether or not I do things perfectly. I confuse my value with my performance.

It's Your Turn

I want you to spend the rest of your session writing your old story. Remember, don't get bogged down by trying to write a pretty story. It doesn't have to be grammatically correct. You can even make up words if you need to. Your goal is simply to express in words how your faulty core beliefs affect the details of your life.

I'll give you one warning here: most people who take this exercise seriously are absolutely shocked by how consistently their core beliefs are driving their stress in multiple areas of their lives. But don't worry if you start to feel overwhelmed by all the stress you are experiencing. Tomorrow you will see why I have encouraged you to invest this time when we begin thinking about how to change your core beliefs. Then, as you begin to become intentional about changing your core beliefs, you'll be ready to create a personalized system that surely will help you live a less-stressed life.

For now, continue to complete your stress log every day. Keep recording your thoughts and feelings three times a day, even if you haven't been stressed. And when you do find yourself stressing out, complete all seven columns of the stress log.

Assignment

- Complete The Old Story About Me worksheet.

- Practice passive or active relaxation for twenty minutes.

- Log thoughts, feelings, and behavior three times a day after breakfast, after lunch, and before bedtime using the stress log.

- Complete all seven columns of the stress log when you *begin* to feel stressed.

THE OLD STORY ABOUT ME

The goal here is for you to understand how your core beliefs play out in the details of your life. Write an autobiography about how people-pleasing, performance, and/or control issues cause you stress in specific relationships, environments, and situations. It doesn't have to be a pretty story, just a short narrative account in which you illustrate the power that the core beliefs have had over your stress process. Use the following guidelines to help you write your story.

My dominant stress-inducing core beliefs center on (check all that apply):

❑ People-pleasing
❑ Performance
❑ Control

My core beliefs have driven my stress in the following areas of my life (check all that apply):

❑ Marriage and family. If so, how?

_____

_____

_____

❑ Work. If so, how?

_____

_____

_____

❏ Self-care (ability to take care of myself). If so, how?

_____

_____

_____

❏ Spiritual life. If so, how?

_____

_____

_____

❏ Friendships. If so, how?

_____

_____

_____

❏ Other areas. If so, how?

_____

_____

_____

The Old Story

❏ Two-sentence summary of my old story

_____

_____

_____

STRESS LOG

This stress log will help you practice becoming more aware of the emotions you experience when your stress begins. It should be completed daily beginning on Day Six of the Stress Relief for Life program. If you encounter a stressful experience during your day, fill out the entire row under the appropriate time period. If you don't have a stressful experience, complete only the first four columns.

	Situation	Thought	Feeling	Behavior	NEW Thought	NEW Feeling	NEW Behavior
Breakfast to Lunch							
Lunch to Dinner							
Dinner to Bedtime							

Day Eleven

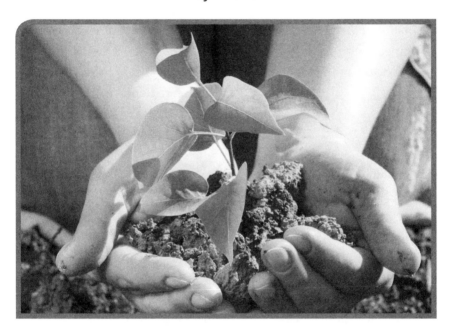

YOUR NEW STORY

LIVE IN FLORIDA or, as we like to call it during the summer and fall, Hurricane Central. I'll never forget the fall of 2004. That's the year my hometown of Cocoa Beach got pounded by three hurricanes in just under two months. The destruction was unbelievable. The day after the last hurricane hit, I decided to ride down A1A on the beachside with my brother-in-law, Mike. The road was covered with probably one foot of sand that had been blown inland from the beach. I exchanged glances with Mike as we passed demolished office buildings and dozens of houses that were in ruins.

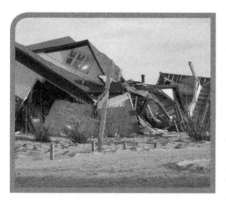

I remember one house distinctly. It sat directly on the ocean and was a classic Florida ranch-style home like the one on the TV show *I Dream of Jeannie*. After the hurricanes, this old ranch seemed utterly lost. The roof had been carried away and every window blown out by the 120-mile-per-hour winds. You could stand on the west side of the house and easily see the waves crashing on the beach through giant openings that used to be windows and doorways.

"This one's a goner," I said to Mike. "There is no recovering from this kind of destruction." I saw no hope that the house could ever be rebuilt and restored to its previous glory.

As I was driving on the same stretch of A1A about a year and a half later, I looked on the site of what was once chaos and destruction and saw a beautiful, stately new home. The builders had retained the foundational footprint of the previous house, but on top of it was one of the most beautiful homes I had ever seen. This was no 1960s Florida ranch; this was a palace. I thought the storm had demolished that old house, but the builders had renewed it to an even greater glory than before.

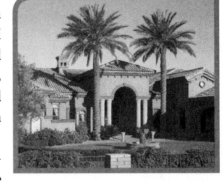

This story has powerful relevance for anyone who is experiencing significant stress. Stress often feels like a storm, and as we've discussed, it can wreak havoc on us physically, relationally, and spiritually. Some of you may feel like you have lived in stress for so long there is no hope that you could ever be renewed or find peace.

But you have a builder who is determined to renew you from the inside out. He intends to bring you to a place that is so far beyond where you were before the storms started, it will exceed your wildest expectations. How? The apostle Paul explains in Romans 12:2 that we are to be transformed by the renewing of our minds.

How is God going to renew your mind? How is He going to transform and empower you to build a life that is less stressed? He is going to start by renewing your beliefs about what makes you acceptable, significant, worthy of connection, and lovable. These core beliefs that drive your hot thoughts are the very mental structures that God wants to transform in your life. And they need to be changed because they are inaccurate.

They are built on what society tells us to value in life. In short, the belief that you can gain significance, worth, or any measure of acceptability by pleasing others, performing well, or controlling things is a lie. It's a lie that the enemy has been feeding your mind since you were too young to know better. And that lie has taken hold and has been directing your hot thoughts in any given situation, environment, or relationship.

Yesterday I asked you to write a story about yourself. The story focused on how people-pleasing, performance, and control issues play out in the details of your life to drive your stress process. It exemplifies the lie about you and demonstrates how the enemy has trapped you in an internal hurricane of stress. From now on we will refer to that story about you, and the underlying stress process that goes with it, in the past tense.

From this moment forth I want you to begin to think about your *real* experience in life as being based on the truth about you—the truth about what makes you acceptable, worthwhile, significant, worthy of connection, and lovable. What's the truth about what makes you OK? On what foundation does a believer base his truth about life, himself, and his worth? Surely the truth about you is based on your status as someone created in God's image. The Bible says God knit you together in your mother's womb.

> For you created my inmost being; you knit me together in my mother's womb. I praise you because I am fearfully and wonderfully made; your works are wonderful, I know that full well.
>
> —PSALM 139:13–14

These verses have tremendous significance for us as believers when understood through the lens of modern science. When the psalmist wrote these words more than twenty-five hundred years ago, he had no knowledge of DNA. But now modern science has identified DNA as the foundation of the human cell and the building block of all that we are as humans. If you look at a model of human DNA, you will see that all our genetic information fits together like a little jigsaw puzzle. Your heavenly Father truly has knit you together.

Of all the combinations of DNA, God chose one for you. You aren't acceptable because other people affirm you or because you're successful or because you can demonstrate good self-control. You're OK because God finds pleasure in you. He doesn't find pleasure in what you do; He finds pleasure in you—period.

"Right, right, right. I get the religious stuff!" That's what many of my clients say when I tell them of the foundation on which they can build the truth about themselves. But they miss the point because this isn't religious at all. This isn't about theological concepts or doctrines. This is about real life at home, at Wal-Mart, during staff meetings, at soccer games, at the grocery store, or wherever.

The problem with the truth about us is that we never give it teeth in our normal, everyday lives. We relegate our status as people who bear God's image, as people in whom He finds pleasure, to our time at church during the worship service. It really is easy to feel like a child of God when we are sharing our faith with the waitress at Denny's, but it's much harder when we feel like we are messing up a relationship. It's easy to feel like someone with whom God finds pleasure when we are singing "O Come Let Us Adore Him" at the Christmas Eve service, but it's much harder when our kids are not being obedient. The key here is to let God's opinion of us saturate every aspect of our experience, even when we aren't feeling very godly. The truth is that we are who God says we are—flaws and all.

Think back to yesterday when you wrote your old story. I asked you to look at how your old core beliefs (note the past tense!) drove your stress in specific situations, environments, and relationships. If you are going to let God renew your mind, to transform the way you think about yourself and your experiences, it is imperative that you cast a vision of how the truth about you impacts very specific aspects of your life. You must get specific about how you can envision giving God pleasure in very real ways.

Your task is to begin to conceptualize the truth about yourself in the details of your life. What is the new story you are going to tell about yourself and how your status as a child of God permeates very specific aspects of your life? You are, perhaps, faced with one of the most awesome and challenging opportunities you have ever had as a person of faith. At the risk of sounding very Oprah-like, you have the chance to reinvent yourself and repair the very spiritual and cognitive structures that have been the source of your stress.

This is a very biblical concept. Jesus Himself said in Mark 8:34, "If anyone would come after me, he must deny himself and take up his cross and follow me." Many people think this verse means you have to deny yourself materially. That might be the case for some, but Jesus's words here are actually even more challenging.

He is encouraging you to deny yourself, to deny the very parts of yourself that define you. Jesus is saying, "If you want to come after Me, you have to give up the parts of yourself that you think lead to your significance, your worth, and your lovability because I'm the only thing you will ever find significance in." The whole idea of "denying" yourself demands that you embrace the truth of your status as God's child.

But before you go off and think you will have to completely change who you are to become less stressed, I want you to remember the house on the beach that I thought was destroyed. If you will recall, the builders had retained the foundational footprint of the previous house. Yes, the new house looked very impressive and elegant, but it was built on the same footprint. As you begin to think about how the truth can take hold in your life, know that God will help you build your new story on the same footprint you have always had.

If you struggle with people pleasing, God will take your heart for people and help you channel that concern for others in healthy directions with proper boundaries. If you are a perfectionist, God will help you understand yourself as someone who strives to do things with excellence but who knows when good enough is good enough. If you have a control-based core belief system, God will help you cast a vision in your heart of a new story in which you are able to effect change in your environment but remain open to the input and opinions of others. God will take what was once a relative weakness and make it your greatest strength. Therefore, as you begin to conceptualize your new story, don't forget your "footprint."

Write Your New Story

Your assignment for the rest of this session is to write your new story based on your new core beliefs about what makes you acceptable, significant, worthwhile, worthy of connection with others, and lovable. Don't worry about making it a nice, neat little paragraph filled with pithy sentences. On the contrary, erase sentences, insert bullets, and do anything else you may have to do to give this story life. I've included a form that will help you think through the different components of your new story. I've also included a modification of Cooper's new story for you to use as an example.

When you feel you have a good idea of what your new story will say, consider typing it out on a computer. This will allow you to easily edit the story as you move forward in the Stress Relief for Life program. Because several days will be devoted to tweaking the new story and making it richer and more detailed, you will definitely need to have some capacity to adjust the content of your new truth.

Tomorrow is a big day because we are going to integrate all the information you have gleaned about yourself so far to create a personalized system of stress management. I hope you know by now what I want you to do in the meantime: continue to log your thoughts and feelings three times a day, even if you haven't been stressed. If you do find yourself stressing out, complete all seven columns of the stress log.

COOPER'S NEW STORY

I used to live life pretty stressed. Before, I was over-focused on my performance and on the outcome of my effort. I thought success would bring me a feeling of worth, significance, and affirmation. But God has revealed to me the truth about who I really am. The truth is that I am a child of God, someone God finds pleasure in. I focus less on the outcome of my efforts and more on the process of my life in general.

Although I still try to do things to the best of my ability, I know that it is my heart that matters, not whether or not I perform well or do things perfectly. At my core, I'm acceptable to God and am worth something in the eyes of other people because of who I am in Christ, not because of what I do.

I love my wife. I love her because she challenges me to focus on the things that really matter, like our marriage. I do the best job I can to meet her needs, but I know that I am not responsible to make her happy. I express my love to her in very tangible ways, such as by taking care of the lawn and washing the cars. But that's not what I focus on in our marriage. My focus is on connecting with her emotionally and creating memories together that we'll remember forever. I even hope we will have a couple of kids one day!

Professionally, I'm a very successful, competent twenty-nine-year-old guy. I have consistently received positive feedback from coworkers and superiors. I try hard to do a good job at the office, but I know that I am a mere mortal and not a superman. I can do the work of only one person, and I'm OK with that. I have the ability to look at a project and know when it is good enough, and I don't stress when something isn't perfect.

I understand that perfection at the office is probably counterproductive. I allow my team the freedom to do their job, and I don't micromanage their every move. When it comes to deadlines, I try my best to meet them. But I know that it's not the end of the world if we miss a deadline here and there. Overall, I'm pretty peaceful at work and confident in my abilities.

Spiritually, I have embraced the whole concept of grace. I understand that God loves me even when I am not producing spiritually. I focus on the process rather than the outcome in my spiritual life too. God and I are doing so well because I know that He loves me because He created me, not because I am a good enough person. I pray, go to worship services, and share my faith consistently not because I feel like I have to but because I want to.

With regard to my appearance, I am comfortable in my own skin. I try hard to take care of my body, and I work out often. But I'm not obsessed with having the perfect body. I know that is impossible. I just do my best to take care of myself and know that my worth is not based on how big my chest gets but on the fact that I am a child of God.

Summary: My worth and my lovability are based on my status as a child of God. I do my best in every area of my life, but I know that I'm OK even when I'm not perfect. I focus on the process, not the outcome.

Assignment

- Write your new story using the provided worksheet as a guide.
- Practice passive or active relaxation for twenty minutes.
- Log thoughts, feelings, and behavior three times a day after breakfast, after lunch, and before bedtime using the stress log.
- Complete all seven columns of the stress log when you *begin* to feel stressed.

THE NEW STORY ABOUT ME

The goal here is to understand how your *new* core beliefs, which are based on God's truth, play out in the details of your life. Write an autobiography about how the truth about you as a child of God minimizes stress and produces peace in specific relationships, environments, and situations. It doesn't have to be a pretty story, just a short narrative account in which you illustrate the power the truth has (or will have) over your stress process. Use the following guidelines to help you write your new story.

What would your life look like if you were able to live God's truth about you in the following situations, environments, and relationships? Include specific examples showing about how you would be less stressed.

Marriage and family

_____

_____

_____

Work

_____

_____

_____

Self-care (ability to take care of myself)

_____

_____

_____

Spiritual life

_____

_____

_____

Friendships

_____

_____

_____

Other areas

_____

_____

_____

STRESS LOG

This stress log will help you practice becoming more aware of the emotions you experience when your stress begins. It should be completed daily beginning on Day Six of the Stress Relief for Life program. If you encounter a stressful experience during your day, fill out the entire row under the appropriate time period. If you don't have a stressful experience, complete only the first four columns.

	Situation	Thought	Feeling	Behavior	NEW Thought	NEW Feeling	NEW Behavior
Breakfast to Lunch							
Lunch to Dinner							
Dinner to Bedtime							

Day Twelve

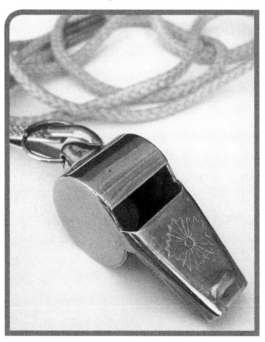

YOUR PERSONALIZED SYSTEM FOR STRESS MANAGEMENT

CONGRATULATIONS! YOU HAVE demonstrated a tremendous amount of diligence to get to Day Twelve of the Stress Relief for Life program. So far you have learned what stress is and where it comes from, and you have become aware of the relationship between your thoughts, feelings, and behavior. You've analyzed which hot thoughts are driving your experience of stress in any given situation, environment, or relationship. You've discovered that your old story is a lie, and you've started to allow God to cast a vision of the new story about you in your heart.

All of this requires time and effort, and I applaud you for having the self-discipline to take the necessary steps to relieve your stress. As I said earlier, if you want the future to be different, you must make changes in the present. And you have. You should be proud of your commitment to yourself and to living a less-stressed life.

On a side note, if you have not given the first eleven days of this program your full attention, I would encourage you to go back and fill in the gaps before you try to forge ahead. Because the program builds on itself, you will likely struggle to create your personal stress-management system unless all the pieces are in place.

If you have completed all the exercises so far, then you are ready to put together all the pieces you've learned to create your personal system for stress management. The beautiful part about creating your personal system is that if you have done all the work up to this point in the program, the transition to your personal system will be seamless. Are you ready to equip yourself to live a less-stressed life? Let's go!

Step One: Stop

You might be wondering why I've had you monitor your thoughts and feelings in the stress logs at least three times a day. Good question. This has been a very intentional assignment because it helped you become more emotionally aware on a moment-by-moment basis.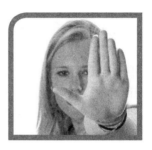
I hope that as you have become more aware of your internal experience, you have been better able to see your stress developing early in the process.

Remember: the earlier you catch yourself in the stress process, the better your chance of stopping your negative response. In short, your assignment has been to start being mindful of your thoughts when you notice yourself becoming stressed. As you complete your personalized program for stress management, continue that process, but also become intentional about suspending whatever you are doing when you catch yourself getting stressed-out. Learning to stop whatever you are doing when you begin to feel stressed is going to take some more discipline. This might even be the hardest part of your personalized system.

One technique that helps many people suspend their activity when they begin to feel stressed is to yell out loud, "Stop." I know this sounds ridiculous, but guess what? It works! There is nothing like yelling to distract yourself from your stress process and give you a clue that you need to refocus. Let me give you a disclaimer here: if you go around yelling stop at the top of your lungs at work or in social settings, you are going to get some funny looks from others. The chances are that your friends, family, and coworkers might not have completed the Stress Relief for Life program, and they might think you are having some fairly serious impulse control problems.

You need a strategy to stop your stress process when others are around that might be less embarrassing than shouting. A more covert strategy that works well is to yell the word *stop* inside your own head. Rather than uttering the word verbally, just yell the word internally.

Let me give you an example here. Have you ever negotiated a deal to buy a car at your local dealership? Remember what you did the first time the salesman returned with his initial numbers? Perhaps you didn't look all that surprised from the outside, but on the inside you were literally yelling, "Are you kidding me?" I'm encouraging the same principle: on the outside, you're cool as a cucumber, a blank slate; on the inside, you're telling yourself very clearly, "Stop!"

For those of you who need a more extreme or physical reminder to stop your stress early in the process, I have one more suggestion. Get a rubber band and start wearing it around your wrist. When you start to feel stressed out, snap the rubber band and yell in your head, "Stop." Needless to say, this small, physical reminder can be extremely effective. After a short training period, the sting of that rubber band will prompt you to stop indulging your stress process and start engaging your personal system.

Is this a rudimentary process? Yes. Is it effective? Very. Should you try it? It's up to you. Perhaps your best option is to try all three methods and see which one works best. At the end of the day, these are just suggestions that might help you unplug from your stress process and begin to implement your personal system for managing stress. Have fun with this, and be creative in your attempts to stop your stress early in the process.

Step Two: Relax

Do you remember when I told you that your personal system for stress management would integrate all the skills we've discussed thus far in the program? Well, we're going all the way back to the passive and active relaxation we learned on days three and 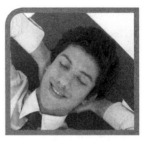 four. After you have disciplined yourself to stop in the early stages of your stress process, you will want to take the edge off of your body's physiological stress response. If you catch yourself early enough in the process, you should be able to relax your body very quickly in the moment.

Now, again, this is contingent upon whether or not you have been diligent in practicing the skills discussed earlier in this program. You are eight days into the relaxation training, and your ability to actually relax your body quickly will only get better the more you practice. Even though you can't relax as well as you will be able to in, say, ten or twelve days, you should already be able to calm down quickly enough to take the edge off physiologically in the moment of your stress.

Obviously, stopping to perform the twenty minutes of relaxation would help anyone who was stressing out. But this isn't quite practical. Can you imagine telling your boss to wait a minute while you spend twenty minutes in the bathroom practicing progressive relaxation? He probably wouldn't get it. Neither would the other people in the bathroom.

The good news here is that you don't need all twenty minutes of relaxation to get the benefit in the moment. On the contrary, after you discipline yourself to stop in the moment, you should be able to take the physiological edge off your stress with just one or two minutes of focused relaxation. That's why you've been practicing this skill every day—the more you practice, the quicker you will be able to get your body into a relaxed state.

Fast-tracking relaxation in one or two minutes is actually simple. Start by taking deep breaths in and out from your diaphragm. This alone may do the trick if you catch yourself early enough in your stress process. You might want to add a second component to this quick relaxation by scanning your body for where the stress seems to be focusing physiologically and then relaxing that specific muscle group. If you find that your neck or back is throbbing, focus in on that muscle group and release the stress just like you do during your practice sessions.

If the active relaxation is more effective for you, flex and relax your neck muscles five or six times while you breathe deeply. If passive relaxation is more effective, relax your neck muscles briefly as you do during your passive relaxation sessions. The important part during step two is to not over-focus on getting the relaxation just right. Your body is not going to feel perfectly relaxed after a minute or two with just eight days of practice under your belt, but you can take the physiological edge off your stress quickly with a little effort during the second step of your personal stress-management program.

Step Three: Think About Your Thoughts

When you've disciplined yourself to stop and relax in the moment, you are ready to start thinking about your thoughts. You've already been doing this while completing your stress logs. Now we are going to add a few new pieces that will make this process even more effective for you.

The hot thought strategy

In step three you should start thinking about your thoughts just as you have earlier in the program. Your first line of defense against the hot thoughts that create stress is still to ask yourself, "Is there another way to look at this situation?" You might want to follow this question with an examination of whether or not your hot thoughts fall into one of the typical categories: all-or-nothing thinking, over-generalization, mental filtering, magnification, globalization, or personalization.

I hope you have already seen how powerful this kind of mental questioning can be to change your perspective and reduce your stress in multiple settings. You have probably also seen how this questioning is incomplete. I have no doubt that you have encountered situations in which simply trying to change the way you are thinking has been ineffective. That's OK. Stress is more complicated than simply changing your hot thoughts about a situation because sometimes your thoughts are rooted more in your core beliefs than in the current situation. If you have more questions about this process, review the reading from the last two days.

The core belief strategy

As you focus in on your thoughts in step three of your stress-management system, there will be times when you will have to work on the level of the core belief to combat your stress. In order to address your stress on the core belief level, start to ask yourself where the hot thoughts are coming from. Ask yourself, "Is this hot thought really driven by the old story, by the lie about me?" If you find roots of a particular hot thought in your old story, then begin to ask yourself what the truth about you is in this situation: "What thought would be induced by the new story about me? How would the new story tell me to think about this?"

These questions should cause you to focus on the truth and give you an opportunity to restructure your thoughts away from the lie. Your job is to let the truth saturate your mind so that it can lead to different thoughts in the moment. Your new thoughts will lead to a rejection of the stress and the adoption of new feelings. Then those new feelings will lead to new behaviors. Remember the example of the eight-year-old who said she hated you after you refused to take her to McDonald's for lunch? I've included an illustration of how step three would look in operation if the core belief strategy were used in this situation.

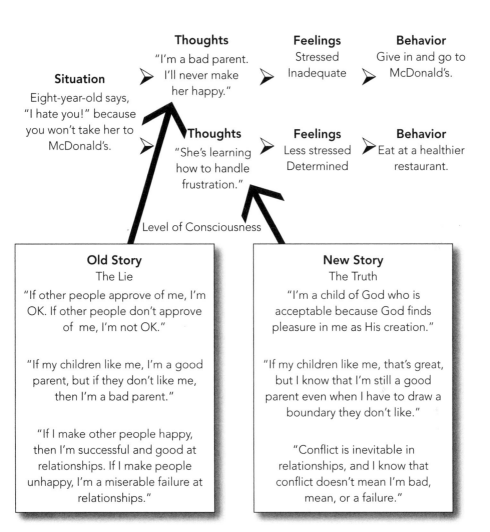

When you start to recognize that your old story is driving your hot thoughts and have considered what the new story would tell you about the situation, you are in a position to begin letting the new story trickle up and saturate your thoughts on a moment-by-moment basis. This is a very difficult process because the thoughts from the old story will seem so normal and comfortable at first. But if you can let the new story saturate your mind when you are stressed to such an extent that you are "thinking on the truth," as the Bible encourages us to do, you will begin to feel much less stressed.

How do you do this? How do you let the truth saturate your mind when the pressure is on? It is hard, no doubt, but it is possible. As you begin this process today, I want you to try something that has worked for many people in the past. Summarize your new story on three-by-five cards that you can place in very conspicuous places—in your car, on your bathroom mirror, and on the refrigerator. Also carry a summary of your new story around with you all day. When a stressful situation arises, pull out your card at the beginning of step three and read the summary over and over. This will allow you to fill your mind with the truth during the stressful situation.

As you do this, it is important to speak the truth aloud. It is one thing to think about the truth and attempt to let it saturate your mind, but it is another thing to speak the truth verbally to allow it to have power in your life. Some of the wisest men who ever lived have confirmed the power of the spoken word. The writer of Proverbs states, "The tongue has the power of life and death" (Prov. 18:21).

Jesus Himself even emphasized the importance of speaking the truth aloud when He told the Pharisees that it's not what goes into the body that's important; it's what comes out of your mouth that either builds up or destroys (Matt. 15:17–18). When you are trying to unplug from the lie and engage the truth, it is important to speak the truth aloud if possible. I know this might not be feasible when you are in a meeting or walking through the mall, but I would encourage you to attempt to find a bit of privacy when you are feeling stressed so that you can take out your three-by-five cards and speak the truth to yourself aloud.

Step Four: Act

After you have aligned your thoughts with the truth about you on the core belief level, you are in a unique position to crush your stress. During step four you are going to put the truth about you into action. Think about what you would do in the stress-inducing 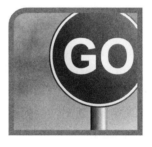 situation if you were completely centered in your new story. Then act in a manner consistent with the new story. Even if you aren't quite feeling like you are able to think on the truth, act as if you are living the truth in that moment. Step four is very important for your stress management over the long term because if you can begin to act in ways that are consistent with the new story, then you will begin to create new experiences that will ultimately confirm the new story.

Let me explain why creating new experiences based on the truth is so important. Remember the example of the eight-year-old who wanted to go to McDonald's? If you were to follow through with your personal system for stress management to the letter, your behavior would be very different from the old story. Rather than taking your child to McDonald's out of guilt, you would go somewhere more appropriate. As you engaged that new behavior, you would more than likely find that your daughter eventually got over her McDonald's fixation and got back to normal.

Depending on how strong your daughter's will is, she might even get over it before you finish with lunch. Then as you are walking out to the car after lunch and your daughter reaches up to hold your hand or gives you a sweet smile, you will start to understand on an emotional level that your worth as a mother or father is not dependent on pleasing your child 24/7. She still loves you, even when you don't do exactly what she wants you to do. The new experience of drawing a boundary with your daughter about junk food will actually end up confirming the new story.

I know this may sound too good to be true. However, it is a fact that when you change your behavior, other people will be forced to adjust the way they respond to you. No, it might not be as seamless as the example above, but ultimately people will have to respond to the new you. As people respond differently to you, you will lay down a new foundation of experiences.

Eventually, as you create a series of new experiences, the new story about you will feel like the real you. Obviously this is a process that will take time to achieve, but the goal of creating change at the core level is very realistic. This kind of change starts with disciplining yourself to make sure that you *act* in accordance with the truth when you are feeling stressed and overwhelmed.

Step 5: Coach Yourself

I hope you are starting to realize that your personal system for managing stress is flexible. After you discipline yourself to stop and relax in a stressful situation, you will be able to see if the hot thought strategy will be sufficient to ease your stress levels or whether you will need to go the extra mile to implement the core belief strategy. No matter how your personal system for managing stress plays out in any given stressful situation, you will want to end with step five.

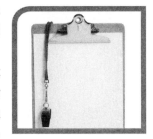

During step five you will implement calming self-talk that will empower you to follow your personal system throughout the entire stressful situation. It is easy to convince yourself during a stressful situation that you are not capable of implementing your personal stress-management system. You will tell yourself things like:

- "This is too much; I can never keep it up."
- "I can't do this anymore."
- "I'll never learn how to manage my stress."

Your goal is to follow through with your entire personal system by making sure that you coach yourself with statements like:

- "This is difficult, but I am coping."
- "I wish my situation were different, but I can make the best of it."
- "My personal system will work if I implement it."

Essentially, step five is just a mental reminder that you are committed to your personal system for managing stress and that the system will work if you use it.

127

My Personalized System for Managing Stress

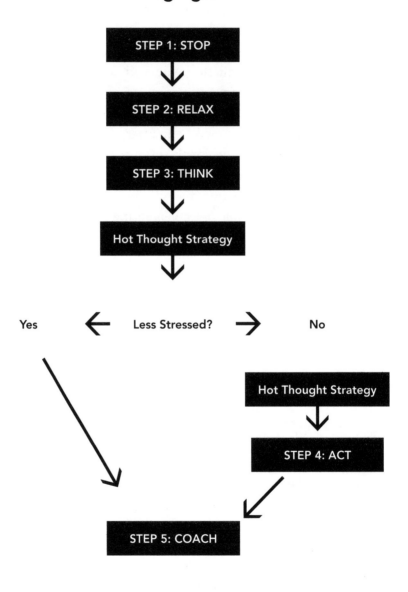

This chart summarizes all five steps of your personal system. It offers all the tools you need to minimize your stress in any given situation, relationship, or environment. Remember, your goal is not to totally eliminate stress from your life. That would not only be unrealistic, but it would also be unhealthy. You're never going to totally eliminate stress because that would make it very difficult to find motivation for the many demands of your life.

Think about it. What if a college student had no stress regarding the upcoming finals? Zero stress about a grade on the test would probably lead to zero studying. Zero studying might even lead to a score of zero on the test. What if a professional basketball player had absolutely no stress regarding his performance during a game? He'd probably be the most passive individual to ever step foot on an NBA court, not to mention the least likely to make it past training camp.

You need a little stress in your life to give you motivation. The purpose of your personal stress-management system is to minimize your stress level in any given situation so that stress isn't a lifestyle for you and you can truly live a less-stressed life.

Consider this day an anchor point in your life. From this day forward, it's go time. You have the skills necessary to crush the stress response in your life. God is going to use your personal system to help you purge the stress-filled life and to reclaim His intention for you: peace—a peace that passes all understanding. So, *go!* Go implement your personal system every chance you get with the assurance that the more you practice these skills, the better you will get at implementing them. The better you get at implementing them, the greater your ability to live a less-stressed life.

I would encourage you to use the rest of today's session to

bathe this process in prayer. You are now more prepared to minimize your stress than you have ever been before, but without the power of God working in your life, you risk continuing to live in the old story. The risk is that you choose to embrace the lie because the truth just seems so hard to live out.

Don't be misled. There are situations that will creep up, maybe even today, that will make your personal system seem very difficult to implement. That is where the power of the Holy Spirit comes in. If you ask God to be present and active in this process for you, He will be faithful to deliver. That is the very nature of God. He is faithful.

I encourage you to end this session by asking for the Holy Spirit's empowerment to implement your personal system and by thanking God for His faithfulness to you in this process. We'll talk more on Day Twenty about how to trust the power of God to sustain all the progress you make in this program. In the meantime, continue to complete your stress log, practice the relaxation techniques, and begin implementing your personal system for stress management.

Assignment

- Pray for the Holy Spirit to empower you to implement your personal stress-management system.

- Practice passive or active relaxation for twenty minutes.

- Log thoughts, feelings, and behavior three times a day after breakfast, after lunch, and before bedtime using the stress log.

- Complete all seven columns of the stress log when you *begin* to feel stressed.

STRESS LOG

This stress log will help you practice becoming more aware of the emotions you experience when your stress begins. It should be completed daily beginning on Day Six of the Stress Relief for Life program. If you encounter a stressful experience during your day, fill out the entire row under the appropriate time period. If you don't have a stressful experience, complete only the first four columns.

	Situation	Thought	Feeling	Behavior	NEW Thought	NEW Feeling	NEW Behavior
Breakfast to Lunch							
Lunch to Dinner							
Dinner to Bedtime							

Day Thirteen

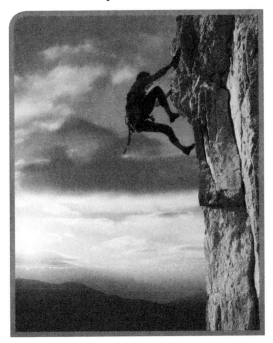

PURSUE STRESS?

HOW IS YOUR personal stress-management system working? I hope you are turning your insights about your stress into action by implementing your personal system in as many situations as possible. Some people get discouraged at this point in the program because they still struggle with significant stress in their lives. If you feel this way, don't worry. Remember, you have all the skills you need to live a less-stressed life, but you must practice them to make the truth a reality.

The more diligent you are to implement your personal system, the more power it will have in your life. If you could fast-forward your life one week, then four weeks, and then four months, you would see the efficacy of your personal system grow and grow. If you continue to implement your personal system, you won't even recognize yourself one day, even when the pressures of life crowd in on you. You'll go from someone who is completely stressed-out to someone who is living the new story.

If you intentionally live the new story in different situations, environments, and relationships, you will start to build a new foundation of experiences. The more you create this new base of experiences, the more the truth will become your standard mode of operation. Pretty soon when you look back on your life, you won't see someone who is struggling with stress and trying diligently to live the truth. Instead you'll see someone who is actually living the new story—someone who is better able to cope with whatever life throws his or her way. Don't be discouraged. Change really is happening!

At this point your job is to consistently create opportunities to implement your personal system so you can develop a foundation of successful stress-management experiences. I know this may sound crazy. You're probably thinking, "Why would I want to create opportunities to be stressed? That's ridiculous!" I definitely understand your concern. Nobody wants to actively seek out stress. Your goal in following this program is to de-stress, not to pursue more stress.

But what if you could implement your personal system during some of your most stressful situations while remaining in a safe and comforting environment? Is that too good to be true? Not really. Researchers have demonstrated over and over again that exposing yourself to significant stress and implementing stress-management techniques in your imagination can be almost as effective as actually experiencing the stress in real life.[1] These imaginary exposure exercises help you to build a new foundation of successful stress-management experiences because they allow you to imagine yourself effectively implementing your personal system in specific stress-inducing situations.

Remember the earlier example in which your pastor unexpectedly asked you to pray during the Sunday morning worship service? You certainly could pursue spontaneous public-speaking opportunities as a way to build a new foundation of experiences in which you successfully implement your personal system. That definitely would work, but it might be hard to actually create this situation. Can you imagine that conversation with your pastor? "Uh...Pastor...if you...uh...ever get the idea that you would like me to pray during the worship service...uh...maybe, don't tell me about it, OK? Surprise me with it. And try to...uh...make it as stressful as possible."

The most stress-inducing situations usually are hard to

create. You can, however, imagine yourself experiencing the stressful event. Athletes do it all the time. Baseball players who are in a hitting slump will imagine themselves hitting base hits over and over again in order to build the confidence to beat the slump. Golfers routinely imagine the ball slowly gliding into the bottom of the hole several times before they actually swing their putter on the green. A basketball player who imagines himself sinking free throws before he steps up to the line is typically a much better shooter than one who doesn't.

We see this principle in Scripture also. If you want to gain the confidence to successfully implement your personal system when the heat is on, it's important to expose yourself to these situations in your imagination first.

Imaginary Exposure

Here's the plan for how you can expose yourself to stress-inducing events without leaving a safe, comfortable environment. Look at the list of your top five stress triggers that you created on Day Five. I want you to focus on number five, the least stressful of the situations or events that stress you out on a consistent basis. Examine the situation and the thoughts, feelings, and behavior it provokes. Next, I want you to close your eyes and begin to implement your relaxation techniques, taking deep breaths and focusing in on the muscle groups where your stress is centering until your body is significantly relaxed. Then imagine yourself encountering the situation you describe in number five of your list.

As you continue to close your eyes and take deep breaths, imagine yourself in this situation in great detail. Imagine which room or environment you would be in as it happens.

You might want to imagine the kind of clothing you would have on, the others who would be present, and what time of day it would likely be. If you think of this situation in enough detail, you will probably begin to feel some slight physiological signs of stress. If that is the case, take a moment and focus on your breathing and relaxation. Don't continue this exercise until you feel a measure of relaxation in your body. If at any time during the remainder of the exercise you begin to notice the physiological manifestation of stress, stop and relax your body.

As you imagine yourself encountering this stressful situation, I want you to imagine yourself implementing your personal system. Imagine yourself successfully thinking about your thoughts. Because you know which hot thoughts are associated with this situation, begin to ask yourself if there is another way to think about the situation. If you need to do so, ask yourself whether your old story is driving the hot thoughts, and imagine yourself replacing thoughts that are consistent with the lie with thoughts that are consistent with the truth.

Now imagine yourself acting in a way that is consistent with the truth about you in this situation. Imagine yourself handling this situation beautifully and experiencing little or no stress as you go through it. Next imagine coaching yourself through this situation, assuring yourself that you have handled it appropriately and that you will handle it appropriately in the future. End this imagery experience with more deep breaths until you feel relaxed and calm.

Depending on how stressful the situation you just imagined was, you might have a real sense of how helpful imaginary exposure can be. Some people find that just imagining an encounter with their fifth most stressful experience creates significant anxiety. If this is the case with you, then imaginary exposure is going to be a very important part of your program. In order to have as much practice with implementing your personal system as possible, over the next four days I want you to practice implementing your personal system for each

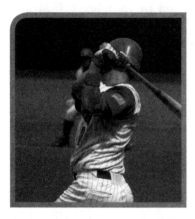

remaining stressor on your list of the top five. This will give you some successful experiences with the situations and environments that are probably going to be the most challenging to your personal system.

After you have practiced managing your stress in all five situations included on your list, you can use imaginary exposure to successfully implement your personal system in any stressful environment or situation. Just like a baseball player who is in a batting slump, use the process I outlined today to imagine yourself successfully implementing your personal system if you find yourself in a "stress slump" in which you are experiencing stress in the same situation over and over again. This is the surest way to build the confidence you will need to successfully implement your personal stress-management system in real-world situations.

Assignment

- Practice passive or active relaxation for twenty minutes.
- Log thoughts, feelings, and behavior three times a day after breakfast, after lunch, and before bedtime using the stress log.
- Complete all seven columns of the stress log and implement your personal system for managing stress when you *begin* to feel stressed.

STRESS LOG

This stress log will help you practice becoming more aware of the emotions you experience when your stress begins. It should be completed daily beginning on Day Six of the Stress Relief for Life program. If you encounter a stressful experience during your day, fill out the entire row under the appropriate time period. If you don't have a stressful experience, complete only the first four columns.

	Situation	Thought	Feeling	Behavior	NEW Thought	NEW Feeling	NEW Behavior
Breakfast to Lunch							
Lunch to Dinner							
Dinner to Bedtime							

Day Fourteen

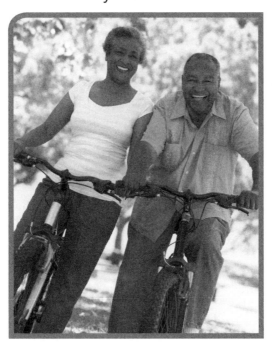

THE POWER OF EXERCISE

I N THE SPRING of 1989 I decided to train to be a beach life-guard. My goal was not to serve the community or to protect helpless swimmers from vicious ocean rip currents. My sole desire was to meet cute girls at the beach—period.

It didn't matter that the other lifeguards-in-training were seasoned, competitive swimmers. I was on a mission to meet the ladies, and not even an exhausting two-mile swim with kids who could swim a mile without breaking a sweat was going to scare me off.

That feeling lasted until about mile marker one. At that point I began to feel an extreme ache in my side and an overwhelming desire to throw up. Hindsight is 20/20, but something tells me that lying on the training pool deck in agony is not all that attractive.

Have you ever exercised so hard you felt like you were going to throw up? Obviously I have. I grew up with the philosophy that if you're going to exercise, you might as well do it right. That meant pushing yourself to the limit of your ability—even to the absolute edge of consciousness at certain points.

That actually was a fine school of thought for me when I was a teenager. In some ways the physical exertion felt good! Our bodies can handle that kind of punishment when we're sixteen, but not so much when we're thirty-six or fifty-six. This is why so many of us end up abandoning exercise as we grow older—because we just can't bring ourselves to the same level of athletic performance (or agony) we once reached. Instead we become armchair quarterbacks: quick to watch people being active but slow to engage in an exercise routine ourselves.

What does this have to do with stress? A lot. Regular exercise has consistently been associated with lower stress levels.[1]

And the beautiful thing is, you don't have to push yourself to the brink of physical exhaustion for the exercise to help reduce stress. Rod Dishman, a professor of exercise science at the University of Georgia, has reviewed more than 250 studies on the effects of physical exercise on stress. He found that whether a person exercises at 80 percent or 40 percent of his capacity, the effect on stress is the same as long as he works out for at least twenty to thirty minutes.[2] In short, there is no correlation between how hard you work out and the stress-reducing benefit you receive.

Do you know what this means? It means that my push-it-to-the-brink philosophy as a teenager was, well, nothing more than a teenage philosophy. The idea that you have to kill yourself to get the stress-reducing benefit of exercise is a myth. You can live a less-stressed life if you simply decide to fit twenty to thirty minutes of exercise into your day. No marathon training here; just moderate exercise such as walking, jogging, bike riding, gardening, or tennis will do the trick. This kind of exercise is very doable, don't you think? The important thing is that you start an exercise routine and that you follow it every day.

Making the Change

OK, now, I need you to promise me one thing. Promise me that you won't get overwhelmed at this point in the Stress Relief for Life program. I know I have asked you to make some significant changes and to carve out a formidable amount of time to start living a less-stressed life. But here's the deal I'll make with you: I'm not going to ask you start an exercise routine today. I know you have a lot on your plate right now, and if this program starts to stress you out, we are really missing the point.

However, I will tell you that exercise is an extremely important part of living a less-stressed life. So if you don't start exercising right now, I want you to consider beginning a moderate exercise routine in exactly one week. You will complete the program in seven days, and at that point you could devote the twenty minutes or so that you've been using to read this book and complete the assignments to exercise.

This will be a seamless transition for you. As you think about beginning your exercise routine, I want you to come up with a plan for implementing it. I've included a worksheet at the end of today's reading that will help you develop your exercise regimen. It includes what I consider the four essential components of any good exercise plan:

1. Reinforcements. Any good exercise plan will include little rewards for following through. Be sure to think of ways you can reinforce yourself daily, weekly, and monthly for complying with your plan. Your self-rewards might look something like this:

   • Daily: "Every day after I exercise I will treat myself to a fat-free mocha from Starbucks."
   • Weekly: "For every week that I follow through with my exercise plan, I will treat myself to a pedicure or lunch with my spouse."

- Monthly: "For every month that I comply with my exercise plan, I will buy myself a new DVD or a new outfit."

2. Persistence. There is no doubt in my mind that you will encounter obstacles as you attempt to formulate and implement your exercise program. For starters, you are going to tell yourself that you just don't have time to sustain an exercise program. Some of you might encounter motivation problems. Others might have trouble determining which kind of exercise to engage in. No matter what may try to prevent you from exercising, you can follow through with your program if you anticipate obstacles and formulate ways to address the resistance beforehand. I've included a section on the worksheet where you can troubleshoot how you will respond to roadblocks you may encounter.

3. Relaxation. A solid body of research has demonstrated a strong link between exercise and relaxation[3]—the same kind of progressive relaxation we discussed during the first week of the program. After you exercise, make sure you reserve time to lie down for a few minutes, close your eyes, and enjoy the floating effect of the endorphins you just released. This will help you get as much stress-busting potential from your exercise program as possible.

4. Fun. No matter what your exercise plan ends up looking like, make sure you engage in activities you enjoy. You'll be much more successful following through on your program if you are doing things you like. By the way, you don't have to perform the same activity every day. If you walk on Monday, ride your bike on Tuesday. If you garden on Wednesday, swim on Thursday. Whatever you do, have fun with it!

Keep Practicing!

As I've mentioned before, the more you practice the skills you are learning through the Stress Relief for Life program, the more power they will have in your life. Today your assignment is twofold. First, I want you to practice exposing yourself to stressor number four from your Top Five Stress Triggers list using the imaginary exposure exercise we discussed yesterday. Second, I want you to create your exercise plan using the worksheet at the end of today's reading.

As you complete your plan, remember that you don't have to schedule marathon training here. Make your exercise doable and fun. At the bottom of the worksheet, you will see a place to sign your name. I want you to sign the sheet only when you are ready to commit to your program. By signing your name, you are promising yourself that you will follow through with the exercise program and your reinforcements. Blessings on you as you think about creating the kind of lifestyle that will lead to a less-stressed life.

Assignment

- Expose yourself to stressor number four on your Top Five Stress Triggers list by completing the imaginary exposure exercise from Day Thirteen.

- Complete the My Exercise Plan worksheet.

- Practice passive or active relaxation for twenty minutes.

- Log thoughts, feelings, and behavior three times a day after breakfast, after lunch, and before bedtime using the stress log.

- Complete all seven columns of the stress log and implement your personal system for managing stress when you *begin* to feel stressed.

My Exercise Plan

I will exercise on the following days:

❑ Sunday   ❑ Tuesday   ❑ Thursday   ❑ Saturday
❑ Monday   ❑ Wednesday   ❑ Friday

I will exercise for _____ minutes every day.

I will complete the following activities during my exercise routine (circle several):

Swim	Walk	Garden	Roller-skate
Run	Bike	Play tennis	Use treadmill
Jog	Use stair stepper	Play basketball	Jump rope
_____	_____	_____	_____
(other)	(other)	(other)	(other)

The potential obstacles to my exercise program are:

Potential Blocks	My Response
_____	_____
_____	_____
_____	_____
_____	_____
_____	_____

I will reward myself for adhering to this program in the following ways:

Daily Rewards: _____

Weekly Rewards: _____

Monthly Rewards: _____

I commit to start this exercise program after I complete the twenty-one-day Stress Relief for Life program, and I will follow through with this exercise plan as outlined above.

_____

Signed

STRESS LOG

This stress log will help you practice becoming more aware of the emotions you experience when your stress begins. It should be completed daily beginning on Day Six of the Stress Relief for Life program. If you encounter a stressful experience during your day, fill out the entire row under the appropriate time period. If you don't have a stressful experience, complete only the first four columns.

	Situation	Thought	Feeling	Behavior	NEW Thought	NEW Feeling	NEW Behavior
Breakfast to Lunch							
Lunch to Dinner							
Dinner to Bedtime							

Day Fifteen

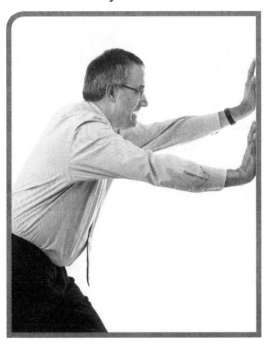

MAKE ROOM FOR MARGIN

'VE GOT A little experiment for you. Look at the following text boxes and consider which one is easier to read and why.

The playwright Jules Renard wrote, "The only man who is really free is the one who can turn down an invitation to dinner without giving any excuse." By that definition, few of us are free. That's a problem. You can't lead a simple life if you can't say no.

The playwright Jules Renard wrote, "The only man who is really free is the one who can turn down an invitation to dinner without giving any excuse." By that definition, few of us are free. That's a problem. You can't lead a simple life if you can't say no.

Although there is some personal preference involved in deciding which text box is easier to read, most people will choose the one on the right because it has wider margins. It's just human nature. When we read through text on a page, most of us prefer some space surrounding the sentences. We like the margins. Look at the page you are reading right now. We could have saved money and printed the text right up to the edge of the page, but we didn't. Why not? Because no one likes to read a book that doesn't have margins around the text. Margins are just more comfortable for us.

The same intuition that leads you to be more comfortable reading a page that has margins leads you to prefer margin in other areas of your life. Having extra space in your life is always more comfortable than living right on the edge. This is true in your financial life, isn't it? Life is more comfortable when you have space in your budget, when you aren't living at the edge of your income every month when you pay your bills. We also pursue margin in relationships. Have you ever asked someone for more space in a dating relationship? That's because relationships can feel smothering if we don't have margin built into them.

Although we need margin in every area of our lives, individuals who are stressed out tend to have very little margin, particularly in their schedules. They don't have any extra space or time to experience the breathing room we all crave. I was struck by this unfortunate reality one day when I was finishing up a counseling session with an eleven-year-old boy. I walked out to the waiting room to make another appointment with his mother, and I whipped out my BlackBerry to see when I had an opening available.

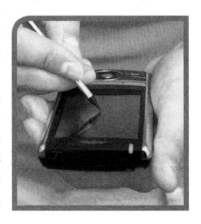

I laughed inside when the client's mother pulled out her own electronic scheduling device to check her calendar. I wasn't really surprised by our little digital scheduling party until something crazy happened right before my eyes. My eleven-year-old client's mother looked at him and asked if he would be available at four o'clock on the next Tuesday. My client immediately pulled out his own handheld device and began to scroll through his appointments. He was more booked up than I was!

Do you see the irony here? When I was eleven, I was riding bicycles and fishing on lazy afternoons after school. This kid needed a PDA just to manage all of his commitments. I bet you can guess why he was in my counseling office in the first place—anxiety. Sure, I'd be anxious too if I were an eleven-year-old boy who had so little margin in my schedule that I needed a handheld device just to manage my daily life.

If a child's schedule can be that full, then imagine the life of the average adult. It's chaos at best. We live life right up to the edge, cramming as much activity as possible into our eighteen-hour days. Why? Because we don't intentionally pursue margin in our schedules, the extra space that will give us time to breathe, relax, and get comfortable.

If you want to live a less-stressed life, it is imperative that you put more margin in your life. Although implementing your personal system for managing stress will surely help in this area, I want you to focus in on two concepts that will help you create more margin in your schedule. If you can master these two principles, you will experience the comfort of having breathing room in your everyday life.

1. Maintain Your Priorities

One reason it is so difficult to create margin in our schedules is that we don't have a true sense of what is most important to us. We want it all—the American dream. The problem is, the American dream has changed in the last several years. We used to be content with having a family, a comfortable home, and a good job. Now we want the kids, the five-thousand-square-foot house, the BMW, the executive position, extensive volunteer activities, an important ministry position in the church, elaborate vacations, and a perfectly toned body.

The problem is, you can't have it all and keep margin in your schedule. It's impossible because the desire for "the dream" will drive you to keep filling your schedule with every opportunity that comes your way. The truth is, no one can maintain more than three or four priorities. If you have a family, that's a priority. If you have faith in God, that should be a priority (emphasis on *should*). If you have a job that you care about, that's a priority.

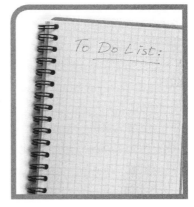

This leaves room for, perhaps, one more priority. Maybe it's staying in shape or volunteering at your child's school—but that's it. Most people understand this intuitively, but they keep overcommitting themselves and overcomplicating their lives. In the process, they destroy any chance they have at experiencing margin in their schedules.

In order to have margin, you must set clear priorities. You must learn how to keep the main thing the main thing. Ask yourself, "What is most important? What do I value most in life?" If you can determine the three or four most important things in your life, then you are in a position to start experiencing some margin. Is this easy? No. Is it necessary? Absolutely. There is no way to create any kind of margin or comfort zone in your schedule unless you are able to focus in on what is essential. Only then will you be able to fill your life with a reasonable number of activities and experience lasting peace and comfort.

2. Learn to Say No

The playwright Jules Renard wrote, "The only man who is really free is the one who can turn down an invitation to dinner without giving any excuse."[1] By that definition, are you free? Few of us are because we feel guilty when we draw boundaries with people in order to focus on what's important. That's a problem. It will be impossible to maintain your priorities and experience margin in your schedule until you get comfortable saying a simple word: no. No excuses, no rain checks, and no babbling about when you might be able to fit it in—just plain no.

Why do we find that so hard as Christians? Why is it so difficult to say no? Probably because on some level we feel that God has called us to be sweet and humble. And we think that sweet, humble people don't deny requests for help and definitely don't turn down invitations to dinner. If this is your struggle, I can't help but point you toward the example of Christ. Yes, He did spend a lot of His time ministering to people—healing the sick, teaching in the synagogues, and sharing the gospel with prostitutes and tax collectors. Yes, He did the ministry thing, and He did it quite well, but He also said no to ministry on occasion.

Take the Last Supper, for instance. On the night before He was to leave this world, we see Jesus spending time with His disciples. He had only a little time left—just a few hours in which to heal the sick, raise the dead, and do ministry—but He didn't spend His final moments that way. He said no to that aspect of His work with people because He knew it was important for Him to be with His disciples at that time. There were also times when Jesus would withdraw from even the twelve disciples just to spend time alone praying, reflecting, and even enjoying nature. In those moments, Jesus was saying no to all the other opportunities He had so He could step back and smell the roses.

Jesus was willing to say no in order to create some margin in His life. Are you? Are you willing to, perhaps, disappoint people when you say no so that you can keep the main thing the main thing? If drawing boundaries or maintaining your priorities has been a problem for you in the past, this might be an issue you'd want to take up in your new story. You can address the concept of creating margin from the perspective of the truth about you.

Remember, your new story is a fluid concept; add a whole new section if you need to. That way you will be able to use your new story as part of your personal stress management system to help you create margin in your schedule on a consistent basis.

Your assignment for today is to get intentional about creating margin in your schedule by maintaining your priorities. I've included a worksheet titled Keeping the Main Thing the Main Thing at the end of today's reading. This will help you think through your priorities and determine whether you are currently committed to activities that are keeping you from creating margin in your schedule. Your assignment tomorrow will help you follow up on the margin you begin to create today.

As you complete both assignments, consider the life of Christ as a model for your own behavior, and ask yourself whether your schedule maintains a healthy balance between ministry, relationships with others, and care for yourself.

Assignment

- Complete the Keeping the Main Thing the Main Thing worksheet.
- Expose yourself to stressor number three on your Top Five Stress Triggers list by completing the imaginary exposure exercise from Day Thirteen.
- Practice passive or active relaxation for twenty minutes.
- Log thoughts, feelings, and behavior three times a day after breakfast, after lunch, and before bedtime using the stress log.
- Complete all seven columns of the stress log and implement your personal system for managing stress when you *begin* to feel stressed.

KEEPING THE MAIN THING
THE MAIN THING

If you want to create margin in your schedule, complete the following steps:

1. Make a list of three or four of the most important things in your life. What would you choose to fill your schedule with? What are the main things?

_____

_____

_____

_____

2. Now make a list of all the things that currently fill up your schedule on a consistent basis. Include everything you are committed to—such as church services, your children's soccer games, work, meetings, volunteer activities, hobbies, school, working out, ministry activities, small groups, etc.

_____

_____

_____

_____

3. Is there an inconsistency between what you prioritize in theory and what you actually spend your time doing? If so, go through your list in question number two and scratch out activities you could eliminate from your schedule. These would be commitments that are not truly priorities for you based on your answer to the first question.

4. Make a commitment to slowly wean yourself off your hectic schedule. Start by cutting out one activity immediately. Then every month remove an activity from your schedule that is not a priority until the only items left are the ones you listed as your true priorities.

STRESS LOG

This stress log will help you practice becoming more aware of the emotions you experience when your stress begins. It should be completed daily beginning on Day Six of the Stress Relief for Life program. If you encounter a stressful experience during your day, fill out the entire row under the appropriate time period. If you don't have a stressful experience, complete only the first four columns.

	Situation	Thought	Feeling	Behavior	NEW Thought	NEW Feeling	NEW Behavior
Breakfast to Lunch							
Lunch to Dinner							
Dinner to Bedtime							

Day Sixteen

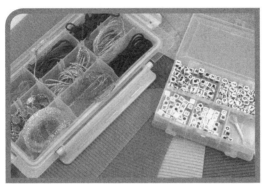

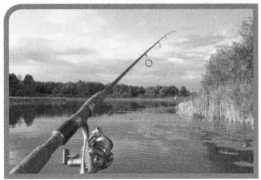

DO WHAT YOU LOVE

Ave you ever seen little children play in a sprinkler? With my adult mind I can't make sense of how it can be so much fun, but apparently this is a pretty huge event in the life of children. They run and jump and frolic with utter joy as they play with a simple sprinkler—a device that represents nothing but work to me. I can't think of anything I like less about yard work than dragging a sprinkler around, turning it on, then running away in an effort to avoid getting drenched. But kids—give them a sprinkler and a warm summer day, and it's on.

Children can have fun in just about any environment. This was demonstrated to me quite dramatically several months ago while I was shopping with my wife at the mall. Now, I'll be the first to admit, walking through the mall is much like watering the lawn for me. I dread it. It was on one of these dreadful trips to the mall that I encountered a young child who was getting dragged around the mall in much the same way I was.

He was probably about four years old, and his mother was in "the shopping zone." She had loaded up her husband's arms with multiple bags from stores like Bath & Body Works, Victoria's Secret, and The Limited. Her husband looked absolutely whipped—for good reason, I'm sure. But this little kid who had been walking around the mall for hours was determined to have fun. I watched him as his dad sank into a chair at one of the women's specialty stores that literally blasts dance music in an effort to make you forget you're spending way too much money on inferior merchandise.

As the thumping rhythm started to invade the little boy's mind, he looked up at his dad, cracked an enormous smile, and then started dancing as if there were no tomorrow. He wasn't a particularly talented dancer; as a matter-of-fact, in another environment one might have thought he was having some sort of seizure. But the kid was having a blast as he threw himself into different positions with utter abandon. As his dad stewed in his own misery, the little boy found a piece of heaven right there in the mall.

What do sprinklers and dancing boys have in common? Well, these two stories demonstrate how willing children are to embrace the fun in life. Without a doubt, kids are masters at finding joy in even the dullest environments. They do what they love to do—what makes them feel alive and free. How often do you do what you really love to do? I'm not talking about sitting in front of the TV watching reruns. I'm talking about doing the things that really nurture your soul, the things that feed your spirit, the things you find exhilarating.

If you're like most people who are overstressed, you don't spend much time doing the things you love—and that's a problem. Researchers have started to identify a new strategy for stress management that has been overlooked for years. Basically, they're finding that one of the easiest and most intuitive ways you can feel less stressed is to engage in activities that you find fun and enjoyable.[1]

Sounds pretty simple, doesn't it? Well, it might be for some people, but having fun is not the typical mode of operation for people who are overstressed. That's why we spent yesterday covering the topic of creating margin. But when you create the needed margin in your schedule, what are you going to do with it? Fill it up with other activities that are stressful? You probably will do just that unless you make an intentional effort to do what you love.

Let's say you work forty hours a week, fifty weeks a year, for fifty years. That's one hundred thousand working hours over the course of your career. One hundred thousand hours of work. How many hours will you spend playing and engaging in the kinds of activities that exhilarate you and make you feel alive? Through the course of your life, the time you spend dancing in malls will probably pale in comparison to the time you spend working.

It makes sense, then, that an important part of managing your stress is to intentionally pursue activities that you find enjoyable. In short, if you're serious about living a less-stressed life, you should cultivate the ability to create margin in your schedule for the things you love, for the things you find exhilarating. You have to become like a child.

Finding Your First Love

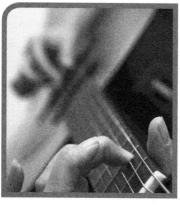One of the biggest problems overstressed people have is that they don't know what they find enjoyable. I can't tell you how many clients I've seen in my practice who can't answer questions such as: What do you like to do? What's fun for you? This happens simply because of the problem stressed-out people have with creating margin in their lives. They are so busy with their chaotic schedules that they don't even have time to consider what they would find exciting or fun.

Can you answer the question: What do you like to do? If

not, it's important that you begin to think about what you can do to have some real fun. One of the best ways to address this in your life is to do what I call a "historical review." Think back over the course of your life about some times when you had great fun. Can you remember a time in your childhood that was distinctly enjoyable? How about in high school or college? Did you have fun playing an instrument? Maybe you can remember a time when you were interested in painting or drawing. Have you ever enjoyed reading? How about scrap-booking or fishing?

The point is, if you can remember times in your life when you had fun, when you felt alive and free, then you should be able to replicate those activities in the present. You are in the process of creating margin in your life. If you can combine your new margin with activities that you truly enjoy, you'll be well on your way to creating a less-stressed life.

For today's assignment I want you to try something very different. Go play in a sprinkler! Metaphorically, that is exactly what I want you to do. Become intentional about embracing play, exhilaration, and enjoyment in your life. Yesterday you thought about how to keep the main thing the main thing as you learned how to create margin in your schedule. Today I want you to cast a vision for yourself of what you're going to do with the time created by your new margin. You can fill it up with more chaos, or you can follow the model of Christ that we talked about yesterday and nurture yourself by engaging environments you find enjoyable. Considering all the work you do, you deserve to have some fun. So check out the worksheet I've included to learn how to do what you love.

Assignment

- Complete the Do What You Love to Do worksheet.

- Expose yourself to stressor number two on your Top Five Stress Triggers list by completing the imaginary exposure exercise from Day Thirteen.

- Practice passive or active relaxation for twenty minutes.

- Log thoughts, feelings, and behavior three times a day after breakfast, after lunch, and before bed-time using the stress log.

- Complete all seven columns of the stress log and implement your personal system for managing stress when you *begin* to feel stressed.

DO WHAT YOU LOVE TO DO

Are you ready to have some fun? As I mentioned in today's reading, new research confirms the truth that engaging in leisure activities we consider fun and exhilarating is an important component of effective stress management. Complete the following exercise to remind yourself of what you really love to do and find exhilarating. Have fun!

1. Perform a historical review in which you think about times/experiences in your life when you've had a tremendous amount of fun. I've included a guide that will help you think this through.

What fun and exciting memories do you have from these times in your life?	
Grade school	
High school	
College	
Adulthood	

2. Based on your past experiences and your knowledge of what you find enjoyable, list several fun activities you could begin to engage in. As you start to free up time in your schedule, enjoy the margin you have created.

_____

_____

_____

_____

3. Remember the little dancing boy? He made what seemed to be a mind-numbingly boring environment exhilarating. Look for opportunities to engage in fun and joy in life even when the situation doesn't necessarily call for it. You might even want to tweak your new story to reflect this concept!

STRESS LOG

This stress log will help you practice becoming more aware of the emotions you experience when your stress begins. It should be completed daily beginning on Day Six of the Stress Relief for Life program. If you encounter a stressful experience during your day, fill out the entire row under the appropriate time period. If you don't have a stressful experience, complete only the first four columns.

	Situation	Thought	Feeling	Behavior	NEW Thought	NEW Feeling	NEW Behavior
Breakfast to Lunch							
Lunch to Dinner							
Dinner to Bedtime							

Day Seventeen

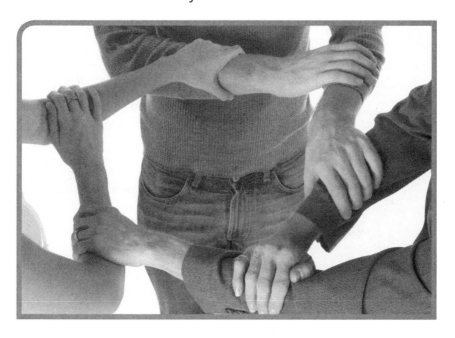

CULTIVATE SUPPORTIVE RELATIONSHIPS

KNEW A GUY when I was in college who was a true free spirit. Conrad couldn't be tied down or restrained, and he certainly didn't have a very good screen on his thoughts. Of course, these traits got him in trouble quite often. But despite his faults, Conrad had a contagious energy for life that could not be denied. When he was around, everyone seemed to have a little more spark. Life seemed a bit more exciting, and the realm of what was possible just seemed to explode.

That's the most impressive thing about Conrad: he brought people to new places. Although he took them to the brink of 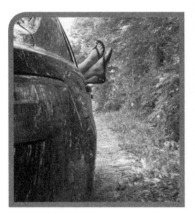 insanity at times, it's fair to say that Conrad moved people. Wherever he went, people had fun. I'll never forget the time Conrad spontaneously decided to drive more than four hundred miles to Atlanta from the University of Central Florida in Orlando. Of course, because Conrad was going, three other guys were immediately interested in tagging along. They loaded up in his car and drove to Atlanta and back in about twenty hours.

Did it make sense? No. Did they have blast? Yes. Those guys are probably still talking about how much fun they had on that trip—all because Conrad was the kind of guy who facilitated a new experience for them, the kind of guy who had a contagious energy and whom you would want on any road trip or at any party.

You know, we all need a Conrad in our life. Actually, we

need several Conrads—people who have a contagious enthusiasm for life and who want to go with us to new and exciting places on the road trip we are taking through life. Considering the fact that you have committed to de-stress, you are in a unique position to need people—supportive people who will facilitate your movement forward and encourage you to take risks and have new experiences.

Do you have any people in your life like this? Do you know any Conrads? Research on stress management has been demonstrating for years the connection between supportive, empowering relationships and relief from stress.[1] You can't go on this journey to a less-stressed life alone. You need to de-stress within the context of relationships, and you need supportive people in your life to stay less stressed. Although the people you surround yourself with don't necessarily need to be impetuous characters like Conrad, they do need to be willing to push you a little bit to engage in new experiences. They need to be interested in you and supportive. And most of all, they need to be encouraging.

When you start to think about the people you will bring with you on your journey to a less-stressed life, zero in on individuals who are:

Good Communicators

If you want to connect with people who will insulate you from the effects of stress, the first quality you should look for is solid communication skills. Good communication has less to do with talking and more to do with listening. Don't go looking for someone you think is smart and eloquent; look for someone you think is caring and empathetic. Look for someone who has the capacity to zero in on you and what's going on in your life at any given moment. Look for people who talk less than they think, reflect, and respond to your experience.

These folks really aren't all that hard to find. In fact, most women in particular are naturally good listeners. I know that is a sweeping generalization, and it is not true in every case, but this gender difference has been documented numerous times in psychological literature.[2] Let me tell you more about the typical woman's listening habits. First of all, women typically use the language of the heart to communicate. In other words, women focus in on your feelings in a given conversation. They love to hear about your thoughts, emotions, goals, and dreams. I believe this is a God-given, natural tendency for many women—the skill of being wonderfully sensitive to the small things people are saying, feeling, or thinking.

This typical mode of operation for many women is in contrast to the usual communication patterns of most men. Men, as a general rule, are great problem solvers who enjoy facts, figures, and data, but we don't listen very well because we don't care very much for the whole touchy-feely world of emotions. As much as it pains me to say this, guys, a strong body of research suggests that merely expressing your feelings through effective communication can do wonders for diminishing the effects of stress in your body.[3] Although most men probably will never be "Mr. Sensitive," it is important that we develop the capacity to communicate on an emotional level.

In a nutshell, the first thing you want to look for in your Conrad-like relationships is that the individuals have the capacity to listen. Should all these relationships be with a woman so that she can listen and respond well? Not necessarily.

I offered this information on gender differences only to give you insight into the type of people you might want to start targeting, but gender differences don't hold true in every situation. There are some men out there who would be more than willing to listen and respond to your feelings. Your goal is simply to connect with people who will communicate with you on an emotional level by talking less than they think, reflect, and respond to your experience.

Grace Oriented

In addition to being good communicators, the people you bring with you on your journey to become less stressed should be grace oriented. They should be the kind of people who can look beyond what is currently happening to see your potential—who you *almost* are. Even in times when you struggle to implement your personal stress-management system or find yourself living in the old story, your Conrad should be able to treat you like you are actively living the new story. He should be your biggest fan in your continuing effort to pursue a less-stressed life.

This is the way God interacts with you. He looks beyond your failures, shortcomings, and brokenness to see the person you almost are. He loves you for who He knows you will be one day in heaven because of the work of Jesus Christ, not for who you are right now because of your earthly accomplishment or lack thereof. Your Conrad needs to be able to refrain from passing judgment if you waver in a specific relationship or environment and to instead refocus you toward your goal of pursuing a less-stressed life.

Honest

The people you choose to support you in your efforts to live a less-stressed life should be willing to be honest with you. They should be willing to speak the truth in love to you on a consistent basis. At times you will need objective feedback from someone about your progress and be held accountable to follow through with your personal system and your new lifestyle choices over the long haul. Whoever you choose to engage on this level shouldn't be afraid to speak the truth to you, even when it is painful or challenging.

Now, let me be clear: by saying this person must be honest, I don't mean he should be brutal with the truth. In fact, someone who constantly points out the obvious to you in an uncaring manner will probably hinder your efforts to de-stress. You need to connect with one or two people who will couple their very real feedback about your behavior with enormous warmth toward you as a person.

For those of you who have been involved in sports over the course of your life, do you remember which of your coaches was most effective? Most people respond to coaches who empower and challenge them, but not to coaches who degrade and ridicule the team. I had a coach in high school who was very knowledgeable but extremely intense and disrespectful. Although he was, perhaps, one of the most intelligent of all the coaching staff, he was despised by most of the guys he worked with. Why? Because he didn't know how to strike the difficult balance between speaking the truth and communicating honor and respect.

When you look for people who can encourage you in your efforts to live a less-stressed life, make sure they are willing to combine honest feedback and accountability with a deep regard for you as a person.

Finding Your Conrad

It has already been established that supportive, Conrad-like relationships are necessary in order to live the less-stressed life over the long haul. Now, I'm about to challenge you to do a very difficult thing. I want you to begin thinking about how you can actually pursue these kinds of relationships in real life. It's one thing to look at the qualities of good communication, grace, and honesty in the abstract; it's quite another thing to identify these traits in people and ask those individuals to hold you accountable to maintain your goal of pursuing a less-stressed life. The truth is that you really do need a Conrad to support you in this process. Proverbs 27:17 says that one man sharpens another as iron sharpens iron. You need someone to sharpen you as you sustain all the progress you have made as a result of your efforts in this program.

One of the biggest objections I hear to the whole idea of finding people who will support you is the claim that they don't exist. My clients often tell me, "I just don't know anyone who will communicate, extend grace, and be honest with me!" While this might be true, my hunch is that you don't know there are people in your life who could be a Conrad for you.

Many times people who are overstressed don't make the time to engage people on a deep level. The truth is that you don't know whether you have people in your life who are willing to be your Conrad until you get intentional about identifying them. You might have a potential Conrad in your Sunday school class. You might eat lunch next to a potential

Conrad every day. You might even sleep next to your potential Conrad every night. I've included an exercise at the end of today's reading that will help you think through the process of targeting potential Conrads. Blessings on you as you think about who you're going to take with you on your journey to a less-stressed life.

Assignment

- Complete the Finding Supportive Relationships worksheet.

- Practice passive or active relaxation for twenty minutes.

- Expose yourself to stressor number one on your Top Five Stress Triggers list by completing the imaginary exposure exercise from Day Thirteen.

- Log thoughts, feelings, and behavior three times a day after breakfast, after lunch, and before bedtime using the stress log.

- Complete all seven columns of the stress log and implement your personal system for managing stress when you *begin* to feel stressed.

FINDING SUPPORTIVE RELATIONSHIPS

If you are serious about living the less-stressed life over the long haul, it's extremely important to identify people who will support you in this process. Of all the characteristics you can look for in the people who will encourage you, try to focus in on individuals who can communicate well, who will freely extend grace to you, and who will give you honest feedback.

Although it may seem difficult to identify people who have these qualities, you might already have relationships with individuals who can become part of your support system. Complete the following steps to begin the process of finding your supportive relationships.

1. Make a list of the people in your life with whom you feel some sort of deep connection. In addition to your spouse, family members, or old friends, include individuals you can picture yourself opening up to. Remember, these people might not have seemed supportive in the past because often those who are overstressed don't make the time to engage people on a deep level.

   _____

   _____

   _____

   _____

   _____

2. Go back through your list and scratch out anyone who you know from previous experience does not

have the qualities of good communication, grace, or honesty.

3. Of the remaining names, check the ones you feel might have the capacity to support you in your de-stress process. You might not know for sure if an individual is definitely capable of being a support to you. That's OK. You just want to identify the people you think would be most able to communicate with grace and honesty.

4. Of the checked names, circle the three you think would be most supportive.

5. During the next couple of days, make contact with these three people and tell them you are currently making a concerted effort to de-stress. Check to see if they would be willing to ask you about your progress on a regular basis.

6. Choose one of your top three supportive relationships to be an accountability partner who will meet with you once a week for thirty minutes over the next three months. During your meetings, ask the individual to encourage you and hold you accountable to implement the stress-relieving skills you've been learning through this program.

7. Don't be afraid to complete the previous six steps. Yes, one of the people you choose to hold you accountable might not be all that supportive in the end. That's OK. If you find that someone is not able to communicate well, extend grace to you, and give you honest feedback, it's not the end of the world or of the program. Just go through this worksheet again and target someone else. The truth is that the more people who know you are intentionally working on decreasing your stress, the more motivation you will have to follow through with the skills in the long run.

STRESS LOG

This stress log will help you practice becoming more aware of the emotions you experience when your stress begins. It should be completed daily beginning on Day Six of the Stress Relief for Life program. If you encounter a stressful experience during your day, fill out the entire row under the appropriate time period. If you don't have a stressful experience, complete only the first four columns.

	Situation	Thought	Feeling	Behavior	NEW Thought	NEW Feeling	NEW Behavior
Breakfast to Lunch							
Lunch to Dinner							
Dinner to Bedtime							

DAY EIGHTEEN

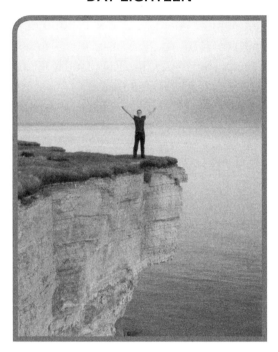

EMBRACE RADICAL CHANGE

CONGRATULATIONS! YOU HAVE exerted a tremendous amount of effort to progress this far in the Stress Relief for Life program. For seventeen days now you have been processing important information about specific stress-management skills and lifestyle changes that will ultimately lead you to a less-stressed life. I know it has taken a remarkable amount of energy and dedication not only to read this book and complete the exercises but also to implement the concepts into your daily life. I applaud your commitment to yourself and to a less-stressed future.

At this point I want to give you a word of advice about how to sustain the progress you have made in the last two and a half weeks. Many people start to experience a very real sense of relief from their stress by implementing their personal stress-management system and engaging the lifestyle changes suggested earlier in the program. I think that by anyone's standards, finding relief from overwhelming stress in just seventeen days is quick progress.

However, the key to seeing results over the long haul is to embrace the changes you have made in your thought life and in your lifestyle beyond the twenty-one days outlined in this book. In short, in order for this program to really have staying power, you are going to need to sustain the changes you have made indefinitely, even in the environments and situations that seem impossible right now. Changing what you do for twenty-one days is one thing. Changing for one year or ten years is quite another.

This is why I've focused your reading for the next three days on the essentials of change. In order to sustain real and lasting change in your thought life and lifestyle, you need to have three strategies in place. Today we'll look at some powerful research that indicates you must embrace radical change consistently in order to sustain the gains you have made so far. Tomorrow I'll point you toward the idea of confronting your fear as a necessary step in the quest to crystallize the progress you have made during the program. Finally, on Day Twenty, we'll discuss the power of the Holy Spirit as the driving force in your change process.

Change or Die?

"Change or die!" What if someone came to you today and made that statement? You'd have only two options: either make changes in your life or bite the dust, pass away, and head home—simply put, die. What would you do? Would you choose to change, or would you choose to die? That's not a hard decision. If we were forced to choose between changing and dying, the natural human reaction would be to choose to change, right?

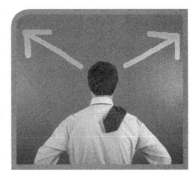

Amazingly enough, for years a specific group of people have been given the choice to change or die, and the overwhelming majority of them choose to die! Staggering, isn't it? Those who have been diagnosed with cardiovascular disease are consistently informed by their physicians after surgery that they will either have to change their lifestyle—their diet, exercise habits, stress-management system, and so on—or they will eventually die. Ultimately, only 10 percent of these patients are able to sustain any real change in their lifestyle; 90 percent choose the option to "die."[1]

Why? Why do so many with cardiovascular disease choose to abandon change and ultimately die from the disease? It has something to do with the scientific community's widely held view of how change happens. Basically, psychologists have done an inordinate amount of research on making and sustaining changes in life. For years they have told people to focus on taking small steps toward change in an effort to slowly approach their larger goals.

So after surgery, those with cardiovascular disease were encouraged to take "baby steps" toward the goal of complete lifestyle change. With regard to exercise, they were encouraged to start by walking slowly for a quarter of a mile each day. With respect to their diet, they were told to make small changes such as cutting out all sweets or reducing their daily calorie intake by 10 percent.

Guess what happened to most of these patients? The small changes in their lifestyle led to disillusionment because they were exercising just enough to make themselves uncomfortable and weren't eating like they used to, but they were losing very little weight and seeing few tangible results.

Finally, someone who worked with these patients got smart. Rather than engaging small steps toward change, these individuals were encouraged to embrace radical, sweeping change. Instead of walking a quarter-mile slowly, the patients worked with a personal trainer to get fit fast. Rather than cutting their calories by 10 percent, they ate tofu and bran flakes. Guess what? More than 70 percent of these cardiovascular patients had sustained their progress three years out.[2]

Why did these patients succeed? Why were they able to choose change over death? Because they were able to immediately reap the benefits of their new lifestyle choices. They experienced the by-products of change in very real ways very early on.

This has important relevance for you. If you are serious about living a less-stressed life, it is essential that you embrace radical change. You can't tiptoe into the new story with an affinity for the old one. You must want to live the truth in every situation, environment, or relationship you engage. It's unrealistic to think that you will live the truth immediately in every area of your life. What's important is that you have a *desire* to live the truth all day, every day.

If you are serious about embracing the lifestyle changes we have talked about throughout this program, it is imperative that you take radical steps in order to sustain those changes over time. You can't take baby steps to implement this program after you have completed all twenty-one days. You can't be content to take small steps in the areas of your life that seem safe. Only when you embrace the new vision of your life fully—with utter abandon—will you experience the staying power of the Stress Relief for Life program. It's only when you embrace sweeping change in every area of your life that you will experience the by-product of change in very real ways.

Go All In

I'm a pretty simple guy, and I do well with basic, real-life examples. Let me tell you how I wrap my brain around the whole concept of embracing radical change. Have you ever seen *World Championship Poker* on some of the obscure cable stations? I used to click right past those stations without even a thought. "Who likes to watch poker on TV?" I thought. "That's like watching pool or bowling on television, or some other 'sport' that no one really cares about."

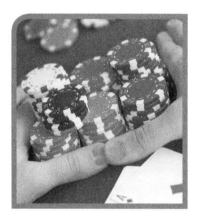

I took this approach until I was up late one night with nothing to watch on TV. It took about thirty seconds for me to realize something about *World Championship Poker*: it is one of the most exciting shows on television! It has interpersonal drama, strategy, risk, and extreme rewards. Somewhere in the midst of my excitement over the game that night, I learned a valuable lesson about both poker and life. At some point, if you are ever going to win at poker, you have to take the risk of pushing all your chips into the center of the table. You have to go "all in," which means you completely commit yourself to the cards you have in your hand at that time. You risk it all for the prospect of winning the prize.

In order to sustain your less-stressed lifestyle, you too must go "all in." You have to completely commit yourself to the vision of a less-stressed life. There's no turning back or reconsidering over the long haul. There's no beating around the bush. You have to embrace radical change, especially in the areas of your life you are most afraid to alter. For some of you, the most problematic area will be that relationship in which the prospect of living the new story is absolutely paralyzing. You have to go all in. For others, it may feel like an impossibility to start an exercise program or to create some margin in your schedule. You have to go all in. Some of you will be scared to death of opening up to someone about your stress process. You have to go all in. If you can discipline yourself to take risks after the Stress Relief for Life program is finished and over with, you will get the prize of a sustainable, less-stressed life.

I'm going to ask you to take a first step toward lasting transformation by getting specific about the areas of your life in which it seems most difficult to embrace radical change. Remember, the goal of the program is to give you information and tools that will lead to a less-stressed life. After you complete the program, there will still be areas of your life in which it will be challenging to implement your personal stress-management system or lifestyle changes. Where will you be tempted to relax your pursuit of a less-stressed life when these twenty-one days are over? In which environments, situations, or relationships will it be most difficult for you to risk everything and go all in?

I've included a worksheet at the end of today's reading titled Going All In. It will help you think through the areas of your life in which you need to consider embracing radical change in order to sustain the progress you've made with this program. Tomorrow we'll discuss one of the most significant stumbling blocks people face as they attempt to embrace radical change: fear.

Assignment

- Complete the Going All In exercise.
- Practice passive or active relaxation for twenty minutes.

- Log thoughts, feelings, and behavior three times a day after breakfast, after lunch, and before bedtime using the stress log.

- Complete all seven columns of the stress log and implement your personal system for managing stress when you *begin* to feel stressed.

GOING ALL IN

After you complete the twenty-one days of the Stress Relief for Life program, you will still encounter areas in which it will be challenging to implement your personal system or engage lifestyle change. In which environments, situations, or relationships do you think it will be most difficult for you to go all in? Answer the following questions to identify these areas with the goal of ensuring that you take big risks and embrace the kind of radical change that will lead to a less-stressed life.

1. Think about which specific environments, situations, or relationships will be the most difficult to live *the truth* in. Pay special attention to areas of your life where you might be hesitant to change and where people might not respond well to your new, less-stressed life.

Specific Relationships	Specific Environments	Specific Situations

2. Think about the lifestyle changes you've been
   encouraged to make. Which seem the most challenging? Is it starting an exercise program or creating margin in your schedule? Perhaps it's the
   whole idea of pursuing supportive relationships.
   Write out which lifestyle changes seem most difficult
   to implement and why.

   _____

   _____

   _____

   _____

3. Look at your answers to questions one and two
   above. These are the areas where you need to focus
   on going all in. These are the places where you
   need to completely commit yourself to the vision
   of a less-stressed life. You might not perform perfectly in these areas, but that's OK. It's not your
   performance that really counts; it's your attitude
   about whether or not you are going to commit to
   the less-stressed life even when it is difficult to do
   so. Consider what is really challenging you based on
   your answers to questions one and two. My hunch
   is that fear is the main reason you are concerned
   about going all in. Don't worry! Day Nineteen is
   devoted to helping you confront your fears.

STRESS LOG

This stress log will help you practice becoming more aware of the emotions you experience when your stress begins. It should be completed daily beginning on Day Six of the Stress Relief for Life program. If you encounter a stressful experience during your day, fill out the entire row under the appropriate time period. If you don't have a stressful experience, complete only the first four columns.

	Situation	Thought	Feeling	Behavior	NEW Thought	NEW Feeling	NEW Behavior
Breakfast to Lunch							
Lunch to Dinner							
Dinner to Bedtime							

Day Nineteen

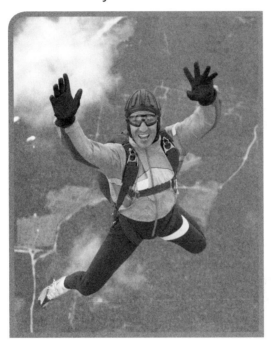

CONFRONT YOUR FEARS

For many of you, the idea of embracing radical change is the most challenging concept you have encountered during this program. If you were paying close attention, you probably noticed that radical change was linked several times with the words *risk, scary,* and *fear.* I must admit that those associations were not accidental.

Here's the funny thing about embracing radical change in your life: the prospect of sliding all our chips to the center of the table and fully committing to a new vision or calling *is* frightening. Being on the verge of committing to the thing God has called us to do is sometimes the scariest place to be on this earth. As you pursue a less-stressed life, you may find yourself downright terrified when you come to the brink of actualizing the peace of God in your life. Why? Because radical change demands that you surrender your comfort zone.

Yes, your stress is disruptive and self-defeating, but it might be a more comfortable place for you. You're used to your stress. That's why you might be tempted to avoid making the tough choices to live the new model and engage the new lifestyle. If you want to live a less-stressed life over the long haul, you have to embrace radical change. And if you want to embrace radical change, you must abandon your comfort zone and confront your fears.

Take the Leap

Many of you reading this book may remember the high dives that used to be a feature at public pools. In case you haven't noticed, most communities don't have high dives anymore because they are such an insurance liability. If you're under eighteen years of age, you probably don't know that we used to jump off platforms that seemed twenty stories high. Now we don't even let our kids dive off the pool deck. I can imagine what a modern mom might say about that: "Now, Johnny, it wouldn't be prudent to do a cannonball; we have to practice pool safety."

But twenty years ago, it was nothing to walk into your local public pool and encounter what seemed to be an enormous tower hovering above even the smallest pool. Conquering the high dive was a rite of passage of sorts. Any boy over the age of four was encouraged to jump off the high dive to demonstrate that he was a risk-taking, adventurous male. To veteran poolgoers, it really didn't matter whether you knew how to swim either: "Oh, you're going up on 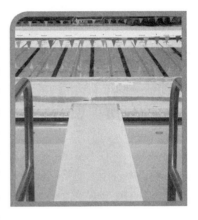 that high dive, Billy? Make sure you take your inner tube. You don't want to sink right to the bottom."

If you're old enough to have seen these dinosaurs, or perhaps to have dived off one, I'm sure you remember the mystique and prominence the high dive carried at the pool. I remember one time in particular when I walked into the pool area as a kid and saw the high dive. I couldn't have been more than eight or nine years old. I was in awe of it. It looked so cool and like so much fun. I knew I would garner respect from both the old and young if I jumped off of it, and I was determined to take the plunge.

I quickly pulled my shirt off, kicked my flip-flops to the

side, and literally ran over several people as I stared toward the heavens—and my destiny. Needless to say, I was exhilarated by the thought of my inaugural jump off the high dive. That is, until I got up to the top and looked down. Then, what I thought would be so much fun became an absolutely terrifying situation.

Have you ever had a similar experience? Do you remember the feeling of being up on a high dive looking down into the water below? It might have seemed twenty stories high from the pool deck, but from the diving platform it suddenly felt like the highest point on Planet Earth. I remember having a sinking feeling in my stomach as I stood above the water with everyone watching and waiting for me to jump.

Then, in a moment of sheer terror, I sat down on the diving platform. I don't know what I was thinking at that moment, but I do know that it would have taken a football team's strength to move me forward off the platform or backward down the ladder. I was sure that I didn't want to jump off, but I was also sure that I didn't want to take the long, humiliating climb down the ladder. Everyone was watching. Everyone was waiting. I was sitting.

I was transported back to my experience on the high dive last summer when I took my four-year-old son swimming at our neighbor's house. Camden was just learning to swim without his "water wings," and I placed him on a small ledge that was maybe two feet off the water.

I jumped into the water myself and began to coach him on how to make a big splash in the pool. As I looked in his face, I saw a familiar gaze from my little boy. He had one of those looks that said, "Dad, you must be absolutely crazy if you think

I'm going to jump off this ledge into that water. I don't have my water wings on, I just learned how to swim, and I'm going to sink right to the bottom. No way. I'm not jumping."

I saw myself in Camden that day. I saw the eight-year-old Michael up on that high dive more than twenty years ago with a look of sheer terror on his face. Camden's position suddenly became very familiar to me, and I had one of those experiences that I very rarely have as a father: I knew exactly what to say. I looked up at him and said, "Come on, buddy; just trust me. I'm right here. You're going to love this. Come on, pal. You don't know how much fun you're going to have. Jump for Daddy. I'll catch you." And then Camden gave me one the most beautiful gifts a son can give his father: he jumped. He trusted me enough to jump.

Many of you are in a place similar to the one Camden was in. You are at the top of a ledge looking down at the waters of peace, but you are scared to death. The prospect of fully embracing the change that is required to live a less-stressed life is absolutely terrifying. You're afraid. You don't know if you can do it, and you feel like you might hit a wall that will make it impossible for you to live in the peace God has for you.

But God is calling you out. He's calling you to surrender the old story and embrace the truth about yourself in every aspect of your life. He's calling you to make the lifestyle choices that will lead to a peace you've never known. He's saying, "Trust Me. I'll never leave you in a situation that is too tough to bear. Trust Daddy."

We are always afraid when faced with the prospect of leaving the comfort zone of our stress and choosing trust over fear, but the only other option is to return to the stressed-out life.

If you aren't going to abandon your comfort zone and embrace radical change, your only other choice is to go backward. I'd hate for you to return to your stress, because going backward in life always makes for a sad story.

We last left eight-year-old Dr. Mike sitting on top of the high dive. That story ends quite tragically from an eight-year-old's perspective. Eventually I climbed back down the ladder. The taunts from the older kids were pretty tough to bear, but I was more disappointed in myself than in anything else. I had finally arrived at the coolest place at the pool, and I ended up going backward down the ladder. Now, as an adult, I know that my experience on the high dive is not all that unusual for a child. High dives are scary, especially for kids. Nonetheless, my feeling of dejection was very real, and I can't forget how awful it felt to climb back down that ladder.

Perhaps there is a message we all can take away from my experience. It never feels good to go backward in life. You've worked really hard to absorb information about how to manage your stress, and you've implemented that information in real life. Now your job is to go forward by fully committing yourself to live out the new story in the areas of your life that scare you the most and to make the lifestyle changes you always thought you could never make.

In which relationships or environments does it frighten you to think about living the truth about you? Do you need to make any lifestyle changes that just "scare you to death"? These fears are the most significant stumbling blocks you'll face as you attempt to embrace radical change.

For yesterday's assignment I had you think through the areas of your life in which you need to consider embracing radical change in order to sustain the progress you've made with this program. Today I've included an exercise that will help you think about how to trust God as you adopt radical change in the environments, relationships, and lifestyle choices that frighten you the most.

Assignment

- Complete the Confront Your Fears worksheet.
- Practice passive or active relaxation for twenty minutes.
- Log thoughts, feelings, and behavior three times a day after breakfast, after lunch, and before bedtime using the stress log.
- Complete all seven columns of the stress log and implement your personal system for managing stress when you *begin* to feel stressed.

CONFRONT YOUR FEARS

Look back at your answers to the Going All In worksheet from Day Eighteen. Think of the environments, situations, and relationships in which you are afraid to take risks. Write your answers in the space provided below.

Next, think of some specific ways you can trust God to help you confront your fears. In particular, think of what God would say to you if He were present in those situations and how He would respond to your fear. Remember, God is asking you to "trust Daddy."

Your Fears	What Would God Say?
Specific relationships: _____ _____	_____ _____ _____
Specific environments: _____ _____	_____ _____ _____
Specific situations: _____ _____	_____ _____ _____
Lifestyle changes: _____ _____	_____ _____

STRESS LOG

This stress log will help you practice becoming more aware of the emotions you experience when your stress begins. It should be completed daily beginning on Day Six of the Stress Relief for Life program. If you encounter a stressful experience during your day, fill out the entire row under the appropriate time period. If you don't have a stressful experience, complete only the first four columns.

	Situation	Thought	Feeling	Behavior	NEW Thought	NEW Feeling	NEW Behavior
Breakfast to Lunch							
Lunch to Dinner							
Dinner to Bedtime							

Day Twenty

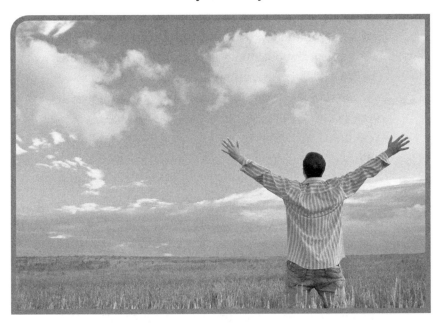

TRUST GOD'S POWER
IN YOUR LIFE

THE STORY OF Jesus's feeding the five thousand is a manual of sorts on how to trust the power of God in your life.

When Jesus heard what had happened to John, he left in a boat and went to a lonely place by himself. But the crowds heard about it and followed him on foot from the towns. When he arrived, he saw a great crowd waiting. He felt sorry for them and healed those who were sick.

When it was evening, his followers came to him and said, "No one lives in this place, and it is already late. Send the people away so they can go to the towns and buy food for themselves."

But Jesus answered, "They don't need to go away. You give them something to eat."

They said to him, "But we have only five loaves of bread and two fish."

Jesus said, "Bring the bread and the fish to me." Then he told the people to sit down on the grass. He took the five loaves and the two fish and, looking to heaven, he thanked God for the food. Jesus divided the bread and gave it to his followers, who gave it to the people. All the people ate and were satisfied. Then the followers filled twelve baskets with the leftover pieces of food. There were about five thousand men there who ate, not counting women and children.

—MATTHEW 14:13–21, NCV

Here we have Jesus and the disciples doing the impossible: feeding more than five thousand people with just two fish and five loaves of bread. Can you imagine what it must have been

like for the disciples in this situation? They must have won-
dered how in the world they managed to be involved in something so amazing. If the truth were told, the disciples didn't
really do anything special to accomplish the miracle. Basically
they passed out bread and fish. That's it. The disciples did what
they knew how to do, and Jesus did what He knew how to do.
The disciples were mere waiters who delivered a meal. Jesus
handled everything else.

The relevance of this miracle for your life is clear. You've
been challenged to make some radical changes, some of which
seem literally impossible. The prospect of living the new story
in the situations that scare you the most or of making the lifestyle changes that will lead to a less-stressed life might seem
pretty far-fetched at this point, kind of like feeding five thousand people with two fish and five loaves of bread. You need to
know that all God expects when you are faced with embracing
radical change is for you to do what you know how to do. He is
responsible for the rest. You do what you know how to do; God
will do what He knows how to do.

You have dedicated the last three weeks to learning some
things you can do to help you live a less-stressed life. You can't
forget to implement what you know how to do. No matter how
stressful life gets or how hard it is to implement your personal
stress-management system, you have to be diligent to con-
tinually put the concepts you have learned into practice. For
example, you can't quit practicing your relaxation exercises or
ignore your personal system when you are in stress-inducing
situations. You can't ignore the information you have received
about creating margin in your schedule, exercising, or finding

supportive relationships. It's essential that you do what you know how to do in order to live a less-stressed life.

If you are willing to be a wise steward of the information you have learned in this program, God will honor your commitment to the less-stressed life, and He will empower you by the Holy Spirit to follow through for the long haul. In the end, a miracle will take place in your life similar to the one the disciples experienced. Trust that. Trust that God will honor your best effort with His miraculous intervention.

Does God really do that? Does He really respond to our best efforts with the miraculous? I can tell you with confidence as a believer myself and as a professional who works with people from all walks of life that God always responds to our faithfulness to do what we know how to do. Sometimes He doesn't respond on the timeline that we would like, but in the end He always rewards our faithfulness with His activity in our life. Your job is to embrace the radical changes this program calls for with a firm awareness that ultimately God will lead you to the less-stressed life. It might not happen tomorrow or next week, but it will happen. You do what you know how to do, and don't quit doing it. God will take care of the rest.

Jason's Story

Jason was a young man with a bright future. He had a good job, was married to a beautiful Christian woman, and was well liked in his community. Jason also had a dirty little secret: he was a methamphetamine addict who had been hooked on the highly addictive drug for two years. During his first visit to my office, he spoke freely about his experience in the grip of meth. He would work for weeks, even months at a time, and maintain all his major responsibilities without a problem. But when he felt meth calling him, his normal existence would cease immediately.

Usually after long, torturous internal battles, Jason would disappear for weeks at a time. He would leave his normal life and enter a crazy drug world that included weeklong parties with people he didn't even know. He described finding himself in strange houses or hotel rooms, high on methamphetamine. Then, as quickly as he had fallen into the trap of meth, he would find his way out. He would drive home and try to undo the damage wrought by his absence.

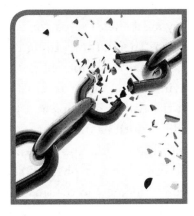

This cycle went on for two long years, and Jason's life was literally falling apart at the seams. His wife was at a loss for how to help him; he couldn't keep a job and was falling deeper in debt.

Early in our counseling sessions we had identified Jason's triggers for relapse. He felt the call of meth when he was stressed out. In a weird way, meth was his coping system for stress. Interestingly enough, Jason continued to struggle with his meth cycles even after he understood the addictive pattern he was in and that his meth use actually caused more stress in the end. He was stuck, and so was I. I had given him all the tools I had at my disposal as a therapist, but Jason was still a meth addict.

Although Jason was close to giving up on himself, his wife refused to concede defeat. She continued to pray, even when Jason went on yet another binge. She begged God to do a work in his life that Jason couldn't do, she couldn't do, and even I, the counselor, couldn't do. Even when she felt like she couldn't go on anymore, she prayed.

Near the tail end of one of Jason's binges, his wife went to church for a prayer meeting. At one point she walked up to the pastor and poured out her heart. Sensing that she was broken beyond belief, the pastor called the whole church to pray for Jason. Then a funny thing happened to Jason.

At that very moment he was lying down on the couch in his living room, about to crash after days without sleep. He was at the end of his rope and was convinced he would be a meth addict until he died. But in those moments God reached down into Jason's life and broke the chains of his addiction. Jason described it as a physical sensation that radiated through his body. He knew in that instance that the power of God had just visited him in a miraculous way.

Until that point, Jason had done everything he knew to do to break free of the grip drugs had on his life. His wife had done everything she knew to do to support him in his recovery. I had done all I could do from a professional stand-point to help him. That's when God came into the picture and honored Jason's heart.

Let me be clear: Jason wasn't done with his share of the work after his experience with God. We continued to meet for months after that to equip him to deal with his stress more effectively. He went to weekly recovery meetings at Narcotics Anonymous, and he started attending church again. But it was encountering the power of God that showed Jason he could be free from his addiction.

God Did It!

Jason eventually beat methamphetamine, one of the most addictive drugs on the streets. But guess what? Jason didn't make this happen, and neither did I as his counselor. Jason just did what he knew how to do. He responded to the call of God in his living room, he came to counseling to learn how to manage his stress, and he went to Narcotics Anonymous meetings. That's it. God did the rest. Jason didn't get himself off meth and into church. God did.

Do you want to live the less-stressed life? If you are ready to embrace radical change by confronting the environments, situations, and lifestyle changes that scare you the most, you have to trust the power of God and expect the miraculous in your life. Twenty days ago you probably couldn't imagine living in the peace of God. You couldn't imagine living a less-stressed life.

But if you continue to practice what you've learned in this program, you'll look back one day and say, "Look what God did. I'm living the life I always dreamed about." And you'll know in those moments that it wasn't you who brought you to peace. If you were totally ready or capable of embracing radical change, you would get the credit, but that's not the point. You'll never be totally prepared to engage the new model in the situations that scare you the most. You'll never be totally ready to implement the lifestyle changes you want to make. You just do what you know how to do. You have the skills now. God will do the rest.

For your assignment today I want you to get intentional about inviting the power of God into your stress-management system. I've included a worksheet that will help you think through this process. I want to encourage you to write a prayer thanking

God for His activity in your life. Get specific by thanking God for helping you embrace radical change in the environments, situations, and relationships in which it seems most difficult to implement your personal system.

I also want you to praise God in advance for empowering you by the Holy Spirit to make the tough lifestyle choices that will enable you to live the less-stressed life over the long haul. I'm asking you to write down your prayer for one very specific reason: it is always helpful to have a written record of what you ask God for. It helps us understand just how faithful He really is and how willing He is to respond to the cries of our hearts.

One day in the future, if you continue to do what you know how to do, you will look down at your prayer and realize that the power of God moved into your stress process and that you are living a miracle. It might happen overnight, or it might develop over a series of weeks, months, or even years. But in the end God's going to do what He knows how to do.

Assignment

- Complete the Inviting the Power of God worksheet.

- Practice passive or active relaxation for twenty minutes.

- Log thoughts, feelings, and behavior three times a day after breakfast, after lunch, and before bedtime using the stress log.

- Complete all seven columns of the stress log and implement your personal system for managing stress when you *begin* to feel stressed.

INVITING THE POWER OF GOD

Use this worksheet to write a prayer to God in which you thank Him in advance for empowering you to embrace the radical change necessary to live a less-stressed life. As you write, be sure to look back at the Going All In exercise so you can be specific about the areas in which you need God to work the most.

After you write your prayer, put it in a prominent place in your house (i.e., on your dresser, the refrigerator, or your bathroom mirror). Every time you see your prayer, thank God again for His very specific activity in your life. Remember, if you are faithful to do what you know how to do, God will be faithful to do what He knows how to do.

MY PRAYER FOR LESS STRESS

STRESS LOG

This stress log will help you practice becoming more aware of the emotions you experience when your stress begins. It should be completed daily beginning on Day Six of the Stress Relief for Life program. If you encounter a stressful experience during your day, fill out the entire row under the appropriate time period. If you don't have a stressful experience, complete only the first four columns.

	Situation	Thought	Feeling	Behavior	NEW Thought	NEW Feeling	NEW Behavior
Breakfast to Lunch							
Lunch to Dinner							
Dinner to Bedtime							

Day Twenty-One

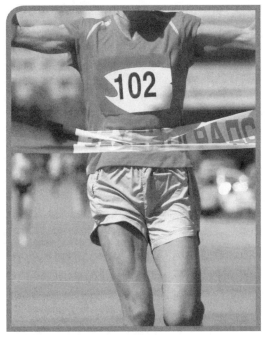

WHATEVER YOU DO, DON'T QUIT

FIRST IMPRESSIONS CAN be hard to shake, can't they? When you picked up this book, you might have thought that when the twenty-one days were over, you could go back to your old lifestyle and still be less stressed. I hope you realize by now that you must implement the skills you've learned indefinitely in order to sustain your progress. Whatever you do, don't quit working the program because you're still at the genesis of a new lifestyle.

To stop doing what you know how to do would be like turning off the engines on a rocket just leaving the launch pad. There's no better way to ensure a crash. If you quit now, you are destined to crash back into chronic stress. It's inevitable. You've just begun a new, less-stressed life. Your job now is to keep flying with your new skills. If you do, you'll eventually find yourself enjoying a life that is full of a peace you have never known.

If you are determined to stay the course to experience a less-stressed life, concentrate on sustaining the following activities.

Relaxation

Your assignments for the last eighteen days has included some form of progressive relaxation because that will help you shut down the stress response in your body. Many people who reach this point in the program rejoice in the fact that they can stop devoting twenty minutes a day to progressive relaxation. Why?

Relaxation is the foundation of a less-stressed life. I concede that you might not have to be as regimented with your relaxation because you want these exercises to serve you— you don't want to serve them. But ultimately you will never be sorry when you devote enough time to consistently and systematically relax your body. Don't quit the relaxation; keep it up on a regular basis to give your body a dose of stress relief.

Your Personal System for Managing Stress

It's easy to get cocky at this point in the program if you are experiencing a marked decline in your stress levels. The more relief you feel from stress, the more likely you are to tune out from your thoughts and feelings on a minute-by-minute basis. No matter how confident you're feeling, don't get sloppy about implementing your personal system for managing stress. It's still incredibly important that you engage your personal system early in any stress process.

Many people ask if it will still be necessary for them to fill out all seven columns on the stress log when they begin to feel stressed. My response is that it varies, depending on the person's comfort level with his personal system. If the individual still struggles to implement his personal system in multiple environments because he isn't quite sure what to do next, the stress log can help him unpack his inner experience. Having an awareness of their thoughts and feelings can help clients implement their personal system with the most efficiency.

My advice to you is to keep filling in all seven columns of the stress log until you are very comfortable cluing in to your inner experience. This will help you implement your personal system with ease and effectiveness.

Radical Lifestyle Change

We have covered at length the benefit of pursuing a lifestyle that includes exercise, creating margin in your schedule, doing what you love to do, and engaging supportive relationships.

Considering the research regarding these matters, it seems clear that in order to sustain the less-stressed life you should pursue all these activities. However, I want you to focus on exercise in particular.

You were encouraged to work out an exercise plan on Day Fourteen. Although there was little pressure to implement your exercise regimen at that time, you committed to yourself that you would start exercising after you completed the Stress Relief for Life program. Well, today is the last day, and there is no better time to start an exercise program than tomorrow. My encouragement to you is simple: take the time you have created in your schedule for this program and use it to complete your exercise routine. Exercising will only move you further along on your journey to a less-stressed life.

Celebrate Good Times, Come On!

Have you ever heard the 1970s hit "Celebration" by Kool & the Gang? From the first "Yeah-hoo," there's something about the song that just makes you want to jump to your feet.

All you have to do is go down to your local karaoke night to

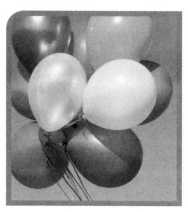

see how powerful this song can be. Most people don't just sing "Celebration"; they experience the song, complete with choreographed dance moves they perform with reckless abandon. There is no doubt: most people get into "Celebration" whenever or wherever they hear it.

Here's the thing that strikes

me as funny: if people were half as good at actually *celebrating* as they are at getting into this song, we would be a lot less stressed as a society. When is the last time you put as much energy into celebrating yourself and what God has done in your life as you can put into singing "Celebration"?

As a general rule, people who have a tendency to be stressed-out don't take much time for celebrating. They don't celebrate themselves, and they don't celebrate God. Stressed-out people are too busy completing the next task on their to-do list to stop and reward themselves for a job well done.

If you are serious about sustaining the less-stressed life, get comfortable with celebration. Celebrate yourself, and celebrate God when you reach milestones in your journey toward the less-stressed life. When you finally live the new story in a scary and difficult environment, do something special for yourself. Go out to dinner or buy a new CD. When you complete your exercise routine for the thirtieth straight day, reward yourself. Buy a new outfit to complement your waning waistline, or take time to call an old friend and just chat.

But most importantly, when you accomplish significant goals that push you toward the less-stressed life, celebrate God. Celebrate His power working in your life and His faithfulness to give you peace. I think it's fair to say that the ability to truly celebrate yourself and God after an accomplishment is diagnostic in nature. It indicates that you are well on your way to living the new story and recognizing how much God loves you. If you are serious about sustaining the less-stressed life, celebrate good times.

As someone who has completed all twenty-one days of the Stress Relief for Life program, you should start celebrating yourself today. You have put a significant amount of energy toward completing this program, and it is worthy of celebration. You deserve to pamper yourself and to love God for giving you the stamina to complete the program.

Today I want you to think of one way you can celebrate yourself for finishing the program. Then think of what you can do to celebrate God because He empowered you to complete all twenty-one days. You can use the worksheet included at the end of today's reading to write out your plan to celebrate your success.

Assignment

- Complete the Celebrate Good Times worksheet.
- Practice passive or active relaxation for twenty minutes.
- Log thoughts, feelings, and behavior three times a day after breakfast, after lunch, and before bedtime using the stress log.
- Complete all seven columns of the stress log and implement your personal system for managing stress when you *begin* to feel stressed.

CELEBRATE GOOD TIMES

Congratulations! You've completed the Stress Relief for Life program. How are you going to celebrate yourself for your commitment to pursue a less-stressed life? What can you do to celebrate God and His commitment to your peace? Write out your plan to celebrate in the space provided below.

Because I am committed to leading a less-stressed life and have completed the Stress Relief for Life Program, I will celebrate myself in the following ways:

_____

_____

_____

_____

_____

_____

_____

Because God is committed to empowering me to live a less-stressed life and because He has enabled me to finish the Stress Relief for Life program, I will celebrate Him in the following ways:

_____

_____

_____

_____

_____

_____

_____

STRESS LOG

This stress log will help you practice becoming more aware of the emotions you experience when your stress begins. It should be completed daily beginning on Day Six of the Stress Relief for Life program. If you encounter a stressful experience during your day, fill out the entire row under the appropriate time period. If you don't have a stressful experience, complete only the first four columns.

	Situation	Thought	Feeling	Behavior	NEW Thought	NEW Feeling	NEW Behavior
Breakfast to Lunch							
Lunch to Dinner							
Dinner to Bedtime							

CONCLUSION

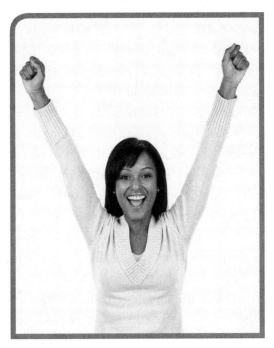

WELL, YOU DID it! You made it through all twenty-one days of the Stress Relief for Life program. One thing is certain: you have demonstrated a tremendous commitment to yourself and to the prospect of living a less-stressed life. My hunch is that you were surprised by the content we have covered in the last three weeks. Who would have guessed that being stressed-out is mostly rooted in lies we've believed about ourselves and that the answer to stress is to free ourselves up to live the truth?

By their very nature, living the new, less-stressed lifestyle and embracing radical change are extremely challenging concepts. The fact that you weren't scared off by the content of this program is a very real indication that you will eventually beat your stress. You are clearly serious about reducing your stress because you are motivated enough to read lengthy information and complete demanding exercises in the hope of eventually living a less-stressed life. If you are reading these words after having completed the program in its entirety, I have great hope that you will find more and more peace in the days ahead.

My hope is that you are already experiencing much less stress. If this is the case, you are tasting the first fruits of a new way of living—a life full of the peace of God that perseveres in the face of any stress-inducing situation, relationship, or environment. If the truth were told, you were never supposed to be stressed-out in the first place. If you remember, at the beginning of the program we talked about how a stressed-out life is a result of the brokenness of our world.

As you continue to act on the information communicated in this book and to implement the skills you have learned, you will find yourself eventually living life the way God intended. Chronic stress is not the way it's supposed to be, but you can live the life you have always dreamed about. Just keep up the hard work. Continue to do what you know how to do, and let God do the rest. Then you'll really be living the dream.

NOTES

Introduction

1. *Grand Canyon*, directed by Lawrence Kasdan (1991; Century City, CA: 20th Century Fox, 1992), DVD.
2. Ibid.

Day One
The Lowdown on Stress

1. Chuck Salter, "Enough Is Enough," FastCompany.com, June 30, 1999, http://www.fastcompany.com/magazine/26/canyonranch.html (accessed January 25, 2011).
2. Mara Der Hovanesian, "Zen and the Art of Corporate Productivity," *Businessweek*, July 28, 2003, http://www.businessweek.com/magazine/content/03_30/b3843076.htm (accessed December 21, 2010).
3. T. H. Holmes and R. H. Rahe, "The Social Readjustment Rating Scale," *Journal of Psychosomatic Research* 11, no. 2 (1967): 213–218. Used by permission.

Day Three
Take Time to Relax: Active Relaxation

1. D. A. Bernstein and T. D. Borkovec, *Progressive Relaxation Training: A Manual for the Helping Professionals* (Champaign, IL: Research Press, 1973); C. R. Carlson and R. H. Hoyle, "Efficacy of Abbreviated Progressive Muscle Relaxation Training: A Quantitative Review of Behavioral Medicine Research," *Journal of Consulting and Clinical Psychology* 61 (December 1993): 1059–1067.

Day Six
Clue In to Your Thoughts and Feelings

1. David Burns, *Feeling Good: The New Mood Therapy* (New York: New American Library, 1980).

Day Thirteen
Pursue Stress?

1. Donald Meichenbaum, *Stress Inoculation Training* (New York: Pergamon Press, 1985).

Day Fourteen
The Power of Exercise

1. K. Hays, *Working It Out: Using Exercise in Psychotherapy* (Washington DC: American Psychological Association, 1999); D. Seymour and K. Black, "Stress in Primary Care Patients," in *Twenty Common Problems in Behavioral*

Health, F. V. DeGruy, W. P. Dickinson, and E. W. Staton, eds. (New York: McGraw-Hill, 2002), 65–87.

2. Matthew P. Herring, Patrick J. O'Connor, and Rodney K. Dishman, "The Effect of Exercise Training on Anxiety Symptoms Among Patients," *Archives of Internal Medicine* 170, no. 4 (February 22, 2010): 321–331.

3. E. S. Sandlund and T. Norlander, "The Effects of Tai Chi Chuan Relaxation and Exercise on Stress Responses and Well-Being: An Overvew of Research," *International Journal of Stress Management* 7 (April 2000): 139–149.

Day Fifteen
Create Margin in Your Schedule

1. ThinkExist.com, "Jules Renard Quotes," http://en.thinkexist.com/quotes/jules_renard/2.html (accessed December 20, 2010).

Day Sixteen
Do What You Love

1. Y. Iwasaki, K. MacKay, and J. Mactavish, "Gender-Based Analysis of Coping With Stress Among Professional Managers: Leisure Coping and Non-Leisure Coping," *Journal of Leisure Research* 37 (2005): 1–28.

Day Seventeen
Cultivate Supportive Relationships

1. S. Haslam, A. O'Brien, J. Jetten, K. Vormedal, and S. Penna, "Taking the Strain: Social Identity, Social Support, and the Experience of Stress," *British Journal of Social Psychology* 44 (2005): 355–370.

2. Deborah Tannen, *Gender and Discourse* (New York: Oxford University Press, 1996).

3. Ibid.

Day Eighteen
Embrace Radical Change

1. Dean Ornish, *Simple Choices, Powerful Changes* (Louisville, CO: Sounds True, Inc., 1998).

2. Ibid.

SELECTED BIBLIOGRAPHY

Bernstein, D. A. and T. D. Borkovec. *Progressive Relaxation: A Manual for the Helping Professionals.* Champaign, IL: Research Press, 1973.

Burns, David. *Feeling Good.* New York: New American Library, 1980.

Carlson, C. R. and R. H. Hoyle. "Efficacy of Abbreviated Progressive Muscle Relaxation Training: A Quantitative Review of Behavioral Medicine Research." *Journal of Consulting and Clinical Psychology* 61 (December 1993).

Haslam, S., A. O'Brien, J. Jetten, K. Vormedal, and S. Penna. "Taking the Strain: Social Identity, Social Support, and the Experience of Stress." *British Journal of Social Psychology* 44 (2005).

Hays, K. *Working It Out: Using Exercise in Psychotherapy.* Washington DC: American Psychological Association, 1999.

Iwasaki, Y., K. MacKay, and J. Mactavish. "Gender-Based Analysis of Coping with Stress Among Professional Managers: Leisure Coping and Non-Leisure Coping." *Journal of Leisure Research* 37 (2005).

Meichenbaum, D. *Stress Inoculation Training.* New York: Pergamon Press, 1985.

Ornish, Dean. *Simple Choices, Powerful Changes.* Louisville, CO: Sounds True, Inc., 1998.

Salter, Chuck. "Enough Is Enough." FastCompany.com. http://www.fastcompany.com/magazine/26/canyonranch.html.

Sandlund, E. S. and T. Norlander. "The Effects of Tai Chi Chuan Relaxation and Exercise on Stress Responses and Well-Being: An Overview of Research." *International Journal of Stress Management* 7 (April 2000).

Seymour, D. and K. Black. "Stress in Primary Care Patients." In *Twenty Common Problems in Behavioral Health.* Edited by F. V. DeGruy, W. P. Dickinson, and E. W. Staton. New York: McGraw-Hill, 2002.

INDEX

A

acceptance 70, 91
accountability 179, 182
addiction 210
adrenaline 8, 25
affirmation 91, 108

B

behavior(s) 11, 18, 44–51, 54, 63–67,
74–75, 82, 86, 96, 110, 116, 122,
125–126, 130, 136, 139, 147, 158,
168, 178, 180, 192, 201, 212, 220

C

cardiovascular disease 187–188
chronic stress 4–5, 9–11, 13, 55, 216,
224
core beliefs
control 25, 55, 73, 77, 81–86,
90–91, 93, 97, 104–105, 107,
118
people pleasing 69, 71–75, 90,
93, 97, 107
performance 77, 79–81,
85–86, 90–95, 97, 104, 108,
129, 142, 193

D

diet 187–188
Dishman, Rod 143
DNA 105

E

Eichling, Philip 9
exercise(s) 12, 18–21, 26, 29, 34, 78,
91, 93, 95, 116, 135, 137, 141–149,
158, 168–169, 180, 186–188, 190–
191, 193, 201, 207, 213, 216–219,
224

F

fear(s) 3, 10, 187, 191, 193, 195–196,
199–202
fight-or-flight 8–9
foundational footprint 103, 107

G

Grand Canyon 3–4

H

hobbies 82, 159
Holy Spirit 130, 187, 208, 212
hot thoughts
all-or-nothing 56, 121
imaginary exposure 135–138,
146, 158, 168, 180
magnification and globalization 57
mental filter 56, 121
overgeneralization 56, 121
personalization 57, 121

K

Kool & the Gang 218

L

Last Supper 156
lifestyle change(s) 186, 188–189, 191–
193, 200, 207, 211, 217

M

margin 151–157, 159, 165–167, 170,
191, 193, 207, 217
McMinn, Mark 3
methamphetamine 208–209, 211

N

Narcotics Anonymous 210–211

National Institute for Occupational Safety and Health 9

P

prayer 80, 91, 130, 210, 212–213
priority(ies) 154–157, 160

R

relaxation
    active 23, 26–29, 34–35, 50, 58, 67, 75, 86, 96, 110, 119–120, 130, 139, 147, 158, 168, 180, 191, 201, 212, 220
    passive 26, 33–40, 120

S

stress, behavioral effect of
    blaming 11
    crying 11
    drinking 11
    eating, increased 11
    fidgeting 11
    nervous habits 11
    pacing 11
    smoking 11
    swearing 11
    yelling 11, 117
stress, emotional effect of
    anger 10
    anxiety 10
    depression 10
    fear 10
    feeling uneven 10
    frustration 10
    impatience 10
    irritability 10
    nervousness 10

short temper 10
worry 10
stress-inducing thoughts 49–50, 54, 56, 61–67
stress management 5, 13, 18, 49, 108, 115–130, 134–135, 138, 157, 165, 169, 175, 177, 186–187, 191, 207, 211
stress, mental effect of
    concentration loss 10
    confusion 11
    indecisiveness 10
    memory loss 10
    sense of humor loss 11
stress, physical symptoms of
    abdominal cramps 10
    chest pains 10
    cold extremities 10
    fatigue 10
    flushing 10
    frequent colds 10
    headaches 10
    heart palpitations 10
    insomnia 10
    muscle aches 10
    muscle stiffness 10
    nausea 10
    sweating 10
    trembling 10
stress, relational effect of 11
stress, spiritual effect of 11
supportive relationships 173–182, 193, 208, 217

T

trust 46, 130, 199, 201–202, 205–212

W

worksheets

Assess Your Stress Level
13–14

Celebrate Good Times 221

Confront Your Fears 202

Creating a Stress-Free Zone
21–22

Do What You Love to Do
169–170

Finding Supportive
Relationships 181–182

Going All In 192–193

Inviting the Power of God 213

Keeping the Main Thing the
Main Thing 159–160

My Exercise Plan 148–149

My Personalized System for
Managing Stress 128

Progress Report From God
91–93

Stress Log 59, 68, 76, 87, 100,
113, 131, 140, 150, 161, 171,
183, 194, 203, 214, 222

The Effects of Stress 15–16

The New Story About Me 111

The Old Story About Me
96–97

Top Five Stress Triggers 51

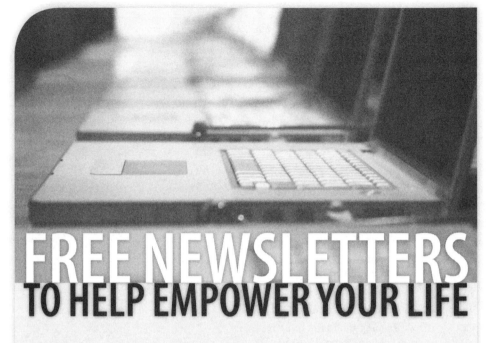